WOMEN'S ISSUES

WOMEN'S PEARLS

WOMEN'S ISSUES

Additional books and e-books in this series can be found on Nova's website under the Series tab.

WOMEN'S ISSUES

WOMEN'S PEARLS

SABINA FINK
AND
PANAGIOTA KORENIS
EDITORS

nova
Medicine & Health
New York

Library of Congress Cataloging-in-Publication Data

ISBN: 978-1-53616-103-8

Published by Nova Science Publishers, Inc. † New York

Dedicated to the most incredibly brilliant and elegant woman I know, My Mother, Rena.

CONTENTS

PREFACE

Women's Pearls is a homage to women, as well as provides clinical pearls written by psychiatrists for clinicians and non-clinicians alike. Mental health as it relates to women is described throughout the chapters of this book. This book represents up-to-date information that can be used as a reference or as a study guide to understand clinical treatment for perinatal mental health. The book demonstrates the history and current understanding of women's mental health. A thorough description of mental health, wellness, diagnosis and treatment recommendations are seen throughout the chapters. Summarized highlights are depicted in each chapter in a form of a table. This book is an excellent learning tool for understanding women's health. It can be used as a self-help book to understand mental health as it relates to women. This book is a review for mental health workers, physicians, residents and students.

ACKNOWLEDGMENTS

This book would not have been possible without the brilliant residents at BronxCare whom had contributed to the chapters. Thank you to my dear co-editor, mentor, and friend Panagiota Korenis. I would like to acknowledge the faculty of my excellent training facility, BronxCare and especially Dr. Korenis and Dr. Shah for their support and encouragement in clinical excellence and education. Most importantly I would especially like to thank my dear parents, grandmother and sisters for their unconditional support and love.

In: Women's Pearls
Editors: S. Fink and P. Korenis
ISBN: 978-1-53616-103-8

Chapter 1

WOMEN

Sabina Fink, MD*
Northwell Health, Garden City Treatment Center,
Garden City, NY, US
Bronx-Care Health System,
Icahn School of Medicine at Mount Sinai, New York, NY, US

INTRODUCTION

Women are like a pearl necklace, each pearl brilliant, beautiful and unique. Over time women have been viewed in different roles, some as daughters, mothers, wives, sisters, physicians, nurses, attorneys, artist, advocates, politicians, and housewives. Many are the backbone, the rock of their own surroundings. Over the years the role has changed for women, from the limitation of only stay at home caretakers, or lower wage earners to full freedom to be anyone they desire to be. However, as the limitless possibilities arise, the balancing act continues. The nature of a woman wanting to be the caretakers never ends. This magnificent amount of multitasking can cause an overwhelming strain on a person. Women

* Corresponding Author's Email: Sfink3@northwell.edu.

sometimes forget to take a minute and evaluate themselves as one that needs to be taken care of. One may need a “me” moment. Self-awareness and wellness is instrumental to maintain a healthy mental state. Women are strong individuals, and many have made instrumental changes in history, history which allows the endless possibilities we now have. Throughout time there have been many great influential leaders and pioneers. From medicine to Hollywood there has been a great change towards equality of women and in praise of women. There are so many great well known female leaders, women whom not only made history, but allowed us to freely choose our paths. Without their passion, strong believes and dedication for equality, many of us would still have less options. There are so many influential ladies in history that’s it’s difficult to name them all. Everyday someone that is making a choice for themselves is paving a way for another young lady looking up to them without them even knowing. Everyone has someone in their lives that has had some sort of positive impact on their paths. As for myself, that is my mother, without whom I wouldn’t have been half the person I am today. For some women it may have been a caretaker, a teacher, a supervising attending, maybe a political figure or a celebrity whom was brave enough to make their voice heard about a personal struggle. Everyday someone might be inspiring someone around them. Many women in this chapter have impacted women of today. It is quiet impossible to name all significant women in history, as there are so many. This book is dedicated to all human beings whom identify as a woman, in celebration of women.

WOMEN IN HISTORY

Dr. Elizabeth Blackwell was the first woman to earn a medical degree in New York in the year 1849. National Women Physician Day (NWPD) is celebrated on February 3rd in honor of Dr. Blackwell’s birthday. The American Medical Women’s Association (AMWA) would like all female physicians across the country to recognize their accomplishments by using social media via hashtags #NWPD and #IAmBlackwell. Dr. Emily

Blackwell was the younger sister of Elizabeth, whom was the third woman to earn a medical degree in the United States.

Dr. Mary Edwards Walker received her medical degree from Syracuse Medical College in New York in 1855. She was a surgeon during the American Civil War, which was considered extremely unusual given the view as women being "unfit" to serve as physicians in the war. She volunteered with the Union Army. Prior to being permitted to work as a physician as she was, she initially had to work as a nurse, before becoming the Army's first female surgeon. While treating wounded soldiers, she was arrested as a prisoner of war, when she crossed enemy lines to assist the ill. Later she received the Medal of Honor. To this day, Dr. Walker is the only woman to receive the Medal of Honor. Dr. Walker was also well known for opposing and refusing to wear traditional female wardrobe. In the 1860's she began to wear what at the time was considered men's clothing. She pioneered in the women's dress reform and she wrote, "The greatest sorrows from which women suffer to-day are those physical, moral, and mental ones that are caused by their unhygienic manner of dressing!" She was a strong voice of the initiation of the women's suffrage movement. Unfortunately, Dr. Walker passed away one year before the 19th Amendment took place.

During the beginning of First World War, of all the physicians only 6% of them were women. Dr. Esther Clayson Pohl Lovejoy whom had stated that "Our Government provided for the enlistment of nurses, but not for women physicians. This was a mistake. It is utterly impossible to leave a large number of well-trained women out of a service in which they belong." Later Dr. Pohl helped establish the American Women's Hospitals Service (AWHS), a program within American Medical Woman's Association which brought humanitarian relief to areas destroyed by war.

Dr. Rebecca Lee Crumpler was the first African American woman to become a physician in the United States. In 1864, she became the first African American graduate of the New England Female Medical School. Same year she married and began a medical practice in Boston. She later wrote a book called "A Book of Medical Discourses in Two Parts," which was published by Cashman, Keating and Co., of Boston, in 1883.

Dr. Gertrude Elion, a daughter to Russian immigrants born in New York was a significant leader in science and medicine. In 1954 she patented a first leukemia-fighting drug "6-mercaptopurine." She received The Nobel Prize in Physiology or Medicine in 1988. She has served as advisor for multiple cancer research projects and committees.

Dr. Mehriban Aliyeva currently holds office as the first Vice-President of Azerbaijan. After completion of school on the highest level in academics with a gold medal, she went on to medical school in Baku, Azerbaijan, subspecializing in ophthalmology in Moscow, Russia. Amongst many of her philanthropic accomplishments including being awarded the title of Goodwill Ambassador of The United Nations Educational, Scientific and Cultural Organization, she has been instrumental in medical, cultural, and political advances in her native country of Azerbaijan. Dr. Aliyeva is not only a philanthropist, physician, a female political pioneer, but also a family oriented woman with an incredible fashion sense.

Women have pioneered throughout history for equality, and ability to achieve great things. Today, we see more women in a multitude of roles. However, there is still room for some improvement in equality. According to the recent Physician Compensation Report of 2019; male physician's earned more than female physicians, as much as 25% higher salaries. This was based on full time employment. The reports also stated that 44% of psychiatrist in the United States are women. Women physicians are leading in the field of Obstetrics and Gynecology, with 61% of positions held by female physicians.

WOMEN OF PSYCHOANALYSIS

The "mothers of psychoanalysis" Helene Deutsch, Karen Horney, Anna Freud, and Melanie Klein as they are referred to in the book by Janet Sayers, were four instrumental women who pioneered to make a significant contribution for women in mental health. They challenged some of the theories that were proclaimed by male experts, and have expanded the field of psychoanalysis.

Helene Deutsch, a patient of Sigmund Freud, reported on her own analysis that she quickly fell in love with her analyst. She was the first woman to lead Vienna Psychoanalytic Society (Sigmund Freud's institute), and she worked on the psychology of women that expanded Freud's work. In the year 1925, Dr. Deutsch published "Psychoanalysis of the Sexual Functions of Women." Dr. Deutsch was the first psychoanalyst to write a book about feminine psychology. Dr. Deutsch later moved to the United States and worked as a psychiatrist at the Massachusetts General Hospital, later she was named the president of the Boston Psychoanalytic Society from 1939 to 1941.

Dr. Karen Horney battled depression from childhood, and at a very young age she decided she wanted to become a physician. This was not an easy task in 19th century Germany. Shortly following graduation, Karen lost both her parents. She entered psychoanalysis to process and deal with her loss. Karen Horney began to work as an analysis in the Berlin Psychoanalytic Society, shortly after she directed the Society's training program. Her roles as female physician, wife, and mother dedicated her to her research on females. Amongst her many contributions to psychoanalysis, Karen Horney challenged the theory of Sigmund Freud's "penis envy" with "womb envy," another words, male envy of woman's ability to have children. Dr. Horney developed the Theory of Neurotic Needs. The theory was broken down to three general categories, one being "Needs that move you towards others," that individuals seek affirmation and acceptance from others; they are clingy as they seek out approval and love. Second category "Needs that move you away from others," the individual creates hostility and are often cold and indifferent. Lastly "Needs that move you against others," the individuals have the neurotic need which result in hostility and a need to control other people, often described as difficult, and or domineering. One of many well stated quotes by Dr. Horney were "there is no good reason why we should not develop and change until the last day we live."

Anna Freud was one of the six children of Dr. Sigmund Freud. As the daughter of Dr. Sigmund Freud, it's no surprise she was interested in psychoanalysis or as her father first called it the "talking cure." However, Anna pioneered in child psychoanalysis and worked extensively on the concept of defense mechanisms to develop ego psychology. Anna Freud earned three honorary degrees from University of Vienna, Jefferson Medical College and Clark University, in Doctor of Medicine, Doctor of Law and Doctorate of Science, respectively. Although, Anna Freud didn't have a formal scientific training per se, she did acknowledge that most of her knowledge came from her home. She declared that while her father had his guest visit, she learned from them. For those of us trained in mental health, wouldn't we all want to be a fly on that wall? Shortly after the Second World War, Anna had opened up The Hampstead War Nursery; this was for orphan children whom had lost their families during the war. The nursery closed in 1952. Following that, Anna Freud opened the Hampstead Child Therapy Course and Clinic, where she was the director. Anna Freud was born in Vienna, Austria, and immigrated along with her parents and siblings to London during the Anti-Jewish movement in the year 1933. She lived in London in their family home until she passed away at the age of 86. During her career, she focused on child psychoanalysis; ego psychology; and childhood development.

Melanie Klein was a psychoanalyst born in Austria, to Jewish Ukrainian- Slovakian parents. Klein is best known for her work on play therapy and the development of object relations theory. Klein believed that children project their feelings in play. As Anna Freud, Melanie Klein did not have formal training. Although she did plan to go to medical school and become a psychiatrist to follow in her father's footsteps, but despite doing well on the entrance exams, she did not have the financial means. Klein married instead for financial stability to support her family following the death of her father. Klein and her family moved to Budapest where she studied psychoanalysis further. There she had met Sigmund Freud. She began to analyze her own children, and following that she published her work "The Development of the Child." While she was in Hungry she had become a member of the Hungarian Psychoanalytic Society. Shortly after she moved to Berlin, then to London secondary to the development of the Anti-Semitic environment. Klein published her book "The Psychoanalysis of Children." Her most well-known paper published was "Notes on Some Schizoid Mechanisms" where she spoke of the relationship of the infant and the mother.

Sabina Spielrein was a Russian physician as well as one of the first female psychoanalysts. Her significances in the beginning stages of psychoanalysis became well known in the 1970's when her diaries and letters were found in Geneva. At a young age she had already learned 4 languages including her native tongue Russian, as well as German, French, and English. Although her parents ensured that Spielrein and her siblings were highly educated including providing them with a governess and a music teacher, the children were in a very strict household including having been beaten by the mother. When Spielrein was 17 years old, her sister died unexpectedly, this caused a lot of distress, and eventually what led her to be admitted to a psychiatric facility for "hysteria" in Zurich where she was the first patient of Dr. Carl Jung. During her stay in the hospital, Spielrein and Jung developed a relationship that would be considered severely unethical given the profession. Much speculation can be raised based on Jung's records, as to what extend the relationship was of a physical nature remains questionable. Following her hospital discharge, she began to attend the University of Zürich to study medicine. In 1911, Spielrein obtained her doctorate. She was elected the second female doctor as a member of the Vienna Psychoanalytic Society in 1911. In the year 1920, Spielrein spoke at the International Psychoanalytic Congress about child development, in attendance was Melanie Klein. Her most well-known work included the treatment of Jean Piaget in 1921 as his analyst. Piaget later developed the theory of cognitive development about the nature and development of human intelligence. Spielrein became director of the child psychology department at the First Moscow University. In 1942 Spielrein was shot along with her children during the catastrophic Nazi attacks on the Jewish people at that time. To this day her life's timeline and events are still being pieced together as her work is still being translated from many languages. A film made in 2011 "A Dangerous

Method" focuses on the relationship between Spielrein, Jung and Sigmund Freud.

Table 1. Women, just to name a few…

Dr. Elizabeth Blackwell	First woman to earn a medical degree in the United States
Dr. Mary Edwards Walker	Only woman to receive the Medal of Honor to date; American Army's first female surgeon
Dr. Esther Clayson Pohl Lovejoy	Helped establish the American Women's Hospitals Service, a program within American Medical Woman's Association
Dr. Rebecca Lee Crumpler	First African American woman to become a physician in the United States
Dr. Gertrude Elion	Recipient of The Nobel Prize in Physiology or Medicine; Patented a first leukemia-fighting drug
Dr. Helene Deutsch	The first woman to lead Vienna Psychoanalytic Society
Dr. Karen Horney	Psychoanalyst, Director of training; Berlin Psychoanalytic Society, Feminine psychology; Theory of neurotic needs; Neo-Freudian psychology
Anna Freud	Psychoanalyst,The Hampstead War Nursery, Hampstead Child Therapy Course and Clinic, Child Psychoanalysis
Melanie Klein	Psychoanalyst, Developed play therapy and the development of object relations theory
Dr. Sabina Spielrein	Psychoanalyst, Director of the child psychology department at the First Moscow University
Susan B. Anthony and Elizabeth Cady Stanton	Leaders of National Woman Suffrage Association
Inez Milholland	Reporter, a suffragist, and a labor attorney
Brook Shields	In 2005, was one of the first celebrities to openly speak about her postpartum depression.
Dr. Mehriban Aliyeva	First Vice President in Azerbaijan, physician, philanthropist, First Lady of Azerbaijan, Goodwill Ambassador.

EVENTS IN HISTORY

The woman suffrage movement, which has initially started in the 1800's, with women getting together, writing petitions and picketing for their right to vote. This movement was what had led to the 19th Amendment, the women's right to vote. It was passed by congress in 1919 and ratified on August 18, 1920. Susan B. Anthony and Elizabeth Cady Stanton, leaders of National Woman Suffrage Association (NWSA) were some of the significant pioneers of this movement. Inez Milholland, was a suffragist, labor lawyer, and a New York Tribune reporter. She was front and center at the women's suffrage march on Pennsylvania Avenue. She was wearing a white cape while seated on a white horse. This event on March 3rd, 1913 overshadowed the inauguration of President Wilson. Milholland died on November 25, 1916 secondary to anemia. Her last words heard in public were, "Mr. President, how long must women wait for liberty?" In the year 1925, in Britain, the woman's rights over her children were granted. Another word, if a biological father wanted to give their child up for adoption, he did not require the permission from the mother to do so. The concept today seems unfathomable. Woman's suffrage was not simply the right to vote, but rather women having rights. Nowadays it's a quick trip to the department of motor vehicle or simply registering online. Incredible women were arrested, ridiculed, and have dedicated years of their lives for this for over a century, so please do exercise your right to vote.

If ever in Salem, Massachusetts, one should visit the Salem Witch Museum, which has a theater portion telling the story of the witch trials, and referring to hysteria quiet frequently. Witchcraft was the crime reported by accusers of the trials. Dr. Quintanilla in her article "Witch Craft or Mental Illness?' described that most plausible differential diagnosis was epilepsy or hysteria as an explanation of what was referred to as witchcraft in Salem. The Salem witch trials lasted from February 1692 to May 1693. Several hundreds of people were accused; some were burned, crushed by stones or imprisoned. Nineteen were found guilty, fourteen of which were women. More were sent to prison and died during their incarceration. As described in the book "Salem Story Reading the Witch Trials of 1692" by Bernard Rosenthal, hysteria was the broadest explanation for the witch trials. One case described by Rosenthal was a women and her deceased child appearing to the accused, as she described her vision in court. Young females, who had suffered from mental illness, sometimes were accused of being frauds in court, or as witches. Physician Ernest Caulfield rationalized 'that they were innocent by reason of hysteria" which was described in Rosenthal's book as "only the outward manifestation of their feeble attempts to escape from their insecure, cruel, depressive Salem Village World."

Table 2. Significant events in history

National Women Physician Day	Is celebrated on February 3rd in honor of Dr. Blackwell's birthday.
The Woman Suffrage Movement.	19th Amendment, the women's right to vote. It was passed by congress in 1919 and ratified on August 18, 1920
The Salem Witch Trials lasted from February 1692 to May 1693.	Several hundreds of people were accused; some were burned, crushed by stones or imprisoned. Nineteen were found guilty, fourteen of which were women.
Women's History Month	Originated in 1982. In 1987 Congress assigned the month of March as "Women's History Month"
International Women's Day	Occurs on March 8th annually by honoring women across the world in majority of countries.
Diagnostic and Statistical Manual of Mental Disorders DSM -III - published in 1980	Was the edition that had removed the diagnosis of hysteria.
Diagnostic and Statistical Manual of Mental Disorders DSM –IV- published in 1994	Added "postpartum onset" specifier
Diagnostic and Statistical Manual of Mental Disorders DSM-V published in 2013	Now used the title "with peripartum onset" which is defined as the most recent episode occurring during pregnancy as well as in the four weeks following delivery.
The U.S. Food and Drug Administration (FDA) have approved the first treatment of postpartum depression on March 19, 2019.	The drug named Zulresso (brexanolone)

March, Women's History Month

Women's History Month had originated in the year 1982. Initially it was a celebration of one week, hence "Women History Week, which began on March 7th. In 1987 after a petition by the National Women's History Project, Congress assigned the month of March as "Women's History Month."

International Women's Day (IWD) is celebrated worldwide on March 8th annually. Today the day is celebrated by honoring women across the world in majority of countries. Why March 8th? March 8, 1857, was when it all began. On that day the employees of New York Garment District protested against long work days, and low wages. The majority of the workers were young female immigrants. The rally was stopped by police, but this led to the first women's labor union. In the year 1908 on the 8th day of March in New York, 15,000 women were marching for better wages

Table 3. Year of women's rights granted by country

New Zealand-1893	China-1949
Australia-1902	India-1950
Finland-1906	Colombia-1954
Norway-1913	Malaysia, Zimbabwe-1957
Denmark-1915	Algeria-1962
Canada-1917	Iran, Morocco-1963
Austria, Germany, Poland, Russia-1918	Libya-1964
Netherlands-1919	Ecuador-1967
United States-1920	Switzerland-1971
Sweden-1921	Bangladesh-1972
Britain, Ireland-1928	Jordan-1974
South Africa-1930	Portugal-1976
Spain-1931	Namibia-1989
Turkey-1934	Western Samoa-1990
France-1944	Kazakhstan, Moldova-1993
Italy-1945	Kuwait-2005
Argentina, Japan, Mexico, Pakistan-1947	United Arab Emirates-2006
Israel, established in 1948- with complete equality of social and political rights to all irrespective of religion, race or sex.	Saudi Arabia-2015

and better hours. Later that year in May 1908, Socialist Party of America stated that the last Sunday in February would be National Women's Day. The first National Women's Day was celebrated on Feb. 28, 1909, in the United States. International Women's Day, was first mention in Copenhagen, Denmark during the international Conference of Working Women. The vote for such celebration was voted by members. No specific date was announced at that point; however several European countries did celebrate in the month of March. The Second Conference of Socialist Women celebrated established March 8 as International Women's Day. How exactly the date was chosen is a speculation of events that were significant enough to pick that date. One theory was the initial gathering in 1857 for better wages, and working environment, and second was a tragic event which occurred coincidently on the same date in 1908. On that day there was an unfortunate event in a fabric factory. One hundred and twenty nine women died in a fire. However the owner of a factory supposedly trapped the women inside so they would not be able to strike with others, and a fire caught in the factory. The fabric that the women were working on was of a lilac hue, which is the color symbolizing IWD. After the women's suffrage during the Soviet Russian Revolution in 1917/1918, IWD was celebrated on March 8th.

Celebrities and Perinatal Mental Health

In popular culture so many celebrities have been open about their own personal struggles of postpartum mood changes. Brook Shields and other celebrities openly spoken about their own illness. Many women face the fear of speaking out about their own struggles with perinatal mood changes. The stigma of what might seem to be "unnatural" of something that is part of many women's nature to be a mother. Despite the social stigma, many celebrity mothers have spoken publicly about the issues they faced surrounding the birth of their baby, as it relates to their mood. Brook Shields in 2005, was one of the first celebrities to openly speak about her postpartum depression, and even wrote a book titled "Down Came the

Rain: My Journey through Postpartum Depression." During an interview with People Magazine, Shields stated "If I had been diagnosed with any other disease, I would have run to get help. I would have worn it like a badge," "I didn't at first - but finally I did fight. I survived." She received a lot of criticism from another celebrity Tom Cruise about her use of anti-depressant following the birth of her daughter. Shortly after many celebrities were coming forward with what they had gone through. Courtney Cox in an interview said "I went through a really hard time - not right after the baby, but when Coco turned six months. I couldn't sleep," "My heart was racing. And I got really depressed. I went to the doctor and found out my hormones had been pummeled." TV star Kendra Wilkinson during one of her interviews in OK magazine talked about her son: "After giving birth, I never brushed my hair, my teeth, or took a shower. I looked in the mirror one day and was really depressed. I thought, 'Look at me!' I had this glamorous life in LA, and now I didn't." Actress Gwyneth Paltrow gave birth to her son in 2006, she later told "Vogue U.K." magazine in an interview: "At my lowest, I was a robot. I just didn't feel anything. I had no maternal instincts for him - it was awful. I couldn't connect, and still, when I look at pictures of him at three months old, I don't remember that time." Many more celebrities came forward and acknowledged their struggles publicly. Many brought awareness to the general public to de-stigmatize the culture of this disease which many struggle with on daily basis throughout a diverse socioeconomic population of women.

HYSTERIA AND BEYOND

The evolution of psychiatry has been a phenomenal force. If we take a look back to "hysteria" to the current edition of the Diagnostic and Statistical Manual of Mental Disorders (DSM), there have been a lot of positive changes. Interestingly enough, hysteria was used as part of a description in a diagnosis until 1980's. Yes, doesn't seem that long ago does it? The DSM III was the edition that has removed the diagnosis of hysteria. The first edition of the Diagnostic and Statistical Manual of

Mental Disorders of the American Psychiatric Association used hysteria as a diagnostic term. The term referred to several presentations including anxiety hysteria, and conversion hysteria.

When you hear someone other than a clinician referring to someone as being hysterical you assume they are being rather expansive in their presentation. Hysteria gets its name from the Ancient Greek word hysteria, meaning uterus. The ancient Egyptians around 1900 BC in the Kahun Papyrus had identified the "hysterical disorders" in women as spontaneous uterus movement within the female body. In the Eber Papyrus around 1600 BC, which is considered the oldest medical document containing depressive syndromes, referenced hysteria to be described as tonic- clonic seizures. Hysteria as it referred to women, was used to describe a wide array of symptomatology including anxiety, fainting, bloating, irritability, and even sexual desire. The uterus was believed to be a "wondering womb" or "hysteria" as described in Ancient Greece by causing incongruent and bizarre presentations in women. Hysteria was also described in 1632 by scientist Edward Jorden, in his book "Suffocation of the Mother." Jorden believed the uterus moved about and caused pressure on the organs, causing an array of unexplained symptoms in women. Hippocrates in the 5th century BC was first to use the term hysteria. Hippocrates too believed that the uterus was a floating organ. Thomas Willis work of hysteria presented that not the uterus, but rather brain and the nervous system were the organs related to hysteria. Post World War Two (WWII), an author by the name of Marion Starkey, had explained that hysteria in young women was aggravated by the intervention of Puritan pastors. This inclined that hysteria could be a consequence of social conflicts. A neuropsychiatrist Pierre Janet, with neurologist Jean-Martin Charcot opened up a clinic in Paris, which proposed hypnosis as treatment of hysteria. Their theory was that the subconscious was the cause of hysteria. Sigmund Freud and Joseph Breuer wrote "Studies on Hysteria" in 1895. The concept of the psychoanalytic theory of the publication evolved around the childhood, sexual fantasies and the different ways of thinking as it relates to the unconscious mind. The original publication of "Studies of Hysteria" may be viewed at the Freud museum located in Vienna, Austria.

Post WWII, there was a decline of "hysteria," and a rise of depression, as suggested by Klerman in 1989.

Many different methods were practiced as treatment of "hysteria." A uterine massage was one way that was believed to treat hysteria. Yes, as much disbelief it brings to a physician today, clinical treatment was used in a form of stimulation to help "treat hysteria." Massaging of a woman's genitals was performed by many health professionals to "cure" via "hysterical paroxysm," or orgasm. An article published in Psychology Today in 2013, explained "By the early 19th century, physician-assisted paroxysm was firmly entrenched in Europe and the U.S. and proved a financial godsend for many doctors." Non-maleficence, the principle of do no harm practiced by physicians comes to mind just imagining these forms of treatments, not to mention the ethical component.

The fourth edition of the Diagnostic and Statistical Manual of Mental Disorders DSM -IV which was released in the year 1994, added postpartum onset as part of diagnostic criteria modifier for other major diagnosis, for example major depression. The specifier was used when symptomology occurred within four weeks of the postpartum period. The DSM-V published in 2013, now used the title "with peripartum onset" which is defined as the most recent episode occurring during pregnancy as well as in the four weeks following delivery. However, untreated peripartum mood and psychosis can persist beyond the four week period.

In recent events, The U.S. Food and Drug Administration (FDA) have approved the first treatment of postpartum depression on March 19, 2019. The drug named Zulresso (brexanolone) injection for intravenous intra-venous (IV) use for the treatment of postpartum depression in adult women. Dr. Tiffany Farchione, the acting director of the Division of Psychiatry Products in the FDA's Center for Drug Evaluation and Research stated in the letter announcing the drug "Postpartum depression is a serious condition that, when severe, can be life-threatening. Women may experience thoughts about harming themselves or harming their child. Postpartum depression can also interfere with the maternal-infant bond. This approval marks the first time a drug has been specifically approved to treat postpartum depression, providing an important new treatment option."

Zulresso is supplied as a solution for intravenous administration. It's administered as a continuous intravenous (IV) infusion over a total of 60 hours (2.5 days) by a health professional, and is monitored for sedation. The efficacy following a four week follow up of Zulresso was shown in two clinical studies in participants who received Zulresso or placebo. The improvement in depression observed was based on depression scales.

There has been a monumental amount of awareness of mental health as it relates to the female sex. The evolution of psychiatry has been captivating!

References

American Medical Women's Association. www.amwa-doc.org (2019) Accessed 3/1/19.

American Psychiatric Association. *Diagnostic and Statistical Manual: Mental Disorders*. 1st ed. American Psychiatric Association; Washington, DC, USA: 1952. [Google Scholar 2019].

American Psychiatric Association. *Diagnostic and Statistical Manual of Mental Disorders*. 2nd ed. American Psychiatric Association; Washington, D.C., USA: 1968 [Google Scholar 2019].

American Psychiatric Association. *Diagnostic and Statistical Manual of Mental Disorders*. 3rd ed. American Psychiatric Association; Washington, DC, USA: 1980 [Google Scholar 2019].

American Psychiatric Association. *Diagnostic and Statistical Manual of Mental Disorders*. 4th ed. American Psychiatric Association; Washington, DC, USA: 2000. [Google Scholar 2019].

American Psychiatric Association. *Diagnostic and Statistical Manual for Mental Disorders*. 5th ed. American Psychiatric Association; Washington, DC, USA: 2013. [Google Scholar 2019].

Castleman, Michael. *Psychology Today* "Hysteria and the Strange History of Vibrators, The invention of the vibrator had nothing to do with women's pleasure". Posted Mar 01, 2013, Accessed 2/2/19.

CBSnews.com. *10 Celebrities Who Battled Postpartum Depression*– Accessed 5/7/19 https://www.cbsnews.com/pictures/10-celebrities-who-battled-postpartum-depression.

Cherry, Kendra, 2019 *Karen Horney's Theory of Neurotic Needs* https://www.verywellmind.com/horneys-list-of-neurotic-needs-2795949 Accessed 1/19/19.

Chodoff, P. 1982. Hysteria and women. *The American Journal of Psychiatry,* 139(5), 545-551.http://dx.doi.org/10.1176/ajp.139.5.545 Accessed 2/1/19.

Cohen, Jennie.2018. *The Medal of Honor: 6 Surprising Facts* https://www.history.com/news/the-medal-of-honor-6-surprising-facts Accessed 5/1/19.

Crann, Sara. 2010. *Profile of Melanie Klein. Psychology's Feminist Voices Multimedia Internet Archive.* Retrieved from http://www.feministvoices.com/melanie-klein/ Accessed 2/19/19.

FDA News Release. *FDA approves first treatment for post-partum depression.* FDA.gov https://www.fda.gov/news-events/press-announcements/fda-approves-first-treatment-post-partum-depression Posted March, 19, 2019, Accessed 5/1/19.

Gul, Pelin. 2010. *Profile of Helene Deutsch. Psychology's Feminist Voices Multimedia Internet Archive.* Retrieved from http://www.feministvoices.com/helene-deutsch/ Accessed 4/1/19.

Hajar, Rachel 2015 "History of Medicine Timeline", *Heart Views.* Jan-Mar; 16 Accessed 3/1/19.

Hall, Karen. "Sabina Spielrein." *Jewish Women: A Comprehensive Historical Encyclopedia.* Jewish Women's Archive. <https://jwa.org/encyclopedia/article/spielrein-sabina>. February, 27 2009, Accessed 2/19/19.

Held, Lisa (2010). *Profile of Karen Horney. Psychology's Feminist Voices* Multimedia Internet Archive. Retrieved from http://www.feministvoices.com/karen-horney/ Accessed 3/1/19.

Kane, Leslie. Medscape.com *Physician Compensation Report 2019.* Posted April 10, 2019, Accessed 4/19/19.

Klein, Melanie. *Trust.* www.melanie-klein-trust.org.uk. Accessed 3/1/19.

Klerman, GL, 1989. Weisman MM. Increasing rates of depression. *JAMA;* 261 Accessed 2/5/19.

Leonard, Elizabeth D. 1994. *Yankee Women: Gender battles in the Civil War*. New York: W.W. Norton & Company. ISBN 0-393-31372-7.

McElvanney, Katie. *Women and the Russian Revolution* https://www.bl.uk/russian-revolution/articles/women-and-the-russian-revolution, the British library Accessed 3/1/19.

Merskey, Harold; Potter, Paul 1989. "The womb lay still in ancient Egypt." *British Journal of Psychiatry.* Accessed 3/1/19.

Nicolosi, Ann Marie. 2007. "The Most Beautiful Sufragette: Inez Milholland and the Political Currency of Beauty." *Journal of the Gilded Age and Progressive Era*, pp 287-310. Accessed 3/11/19.

NobelPrize.org. *Gertrude B. Elion – Biographical.* Nobel Media AB 2019. Wed. 8 May 2019. https://www.nobelprize.org/prizes/medicine/1988/elion/facts/Accessed 5/11/19.

North C. S. 2015. The Classification of Hysteria and Related Disorders: Historical and Phenomenological Considerations. *Behavioral sciences* (Basel, Switzerland).

Quintanilla, Beatriz June 21, 2010. "Witchcraft or Mental Illness?" *Psychiatric times.* https://www.psychiatrictimes.com/schizoaffective/witchcraft-or-mental-illness Accessed 3/1/19.

Rourke, Steven. "Women Physicians Who Changed the Course of American Medicine" *Medscape.com.* February 3, 2017 Accessed 3/1/19.

Shields, Brook. 2006. *Down Came the Rain: My Journey Through Postpartum Depression.* New York: Hyperion.

Smirle, Corinne 2012. *Profile of Anna Freud. Psychology's Feminist Voices.* Multimedia Internet Archive. Retrieved from http://www.feministvoices.com/anna-freud/ Accessed 3/1/19.

Solis, Steph posted Mar 08, 2013. *Where Did International Women's Day Come From?* https://www.yesmagazine.org/people-power/where-did-international-women-s-day-come-from Accessed 3/1/19.

Tasca, C., et al. 2012. *Women and hysteria in the history of mental health. Clinical practice and epidemiology in mental health.*

The First Lady of Azerbaijan. https://mehriban-aliyeva.az/en/ Biography Accessed 5/1/19.

The Library of Congress "March is Women's History Month" https://womenshistorymonth.gov/about/ The Library of Congress Legal USA.gov Accessed 3/1/19.

The Library of Congress. "Profiles: Selected Leaders of the National Woman's Party." *American Memory*. July 19, 2009 Accessed 3/1/19.

The National Constitution Center. https://constitutioncenter.org/interactive-constitution/amendments/ amendment-xix Accessed 3/1/19.

Woolf A. 2000 Witchcraft or mycotoxin? The Salem witch trials. *J Toxicol Clin Toxicol.;* 34:457-460.

In: Women's Pearls
Editors: S. Fink and P. Korenis
ISBN: 978-1-53616-103-8

Chapter 2

ADOLESCENTS AND MENTAL HEALTH

Monica Badillo, MD[*] and Modupe James, MD
Bronx-Care Hospital,
Icahn School of Medicine at Mount Sinai, New York, NY, US

INTRODUCTION

The demand for increasing mental health awareness among adolescents and young adults has become a necessity. With the advent of cyberspace, internet, and increasing access to technology, the host of mental health issues that arise have shown a dramatic increase in recent years. As a result adolescent youths are spending more time utilizing technology and having access to these measures. This chapter will discuss adolescent issues with regards to maturation and development of personality, cyber bullying, sexual behaviors, violence, and suicidality. Sexting also remains an important public health issue as it is associated with increased risk of substance use, risky sexual behavior, cyberbullying,

[*] Corresponding Author's E-mail: mbadillo@bronxleb.or.

and reputational damage. This chapter will also review the topic of adolescent substance use, and the role of adolescent peer pressure.

PHYSICAL, PSYCHOLOGICAL, AND PERSONALITY DEVELOPMENT OF ADOLESCENCE

Adolescence period is a transitional stage of physical and psychological development that occurs during the period from puberty to legal adulthood. Biologically age is used as a rough marker of adolescence, and it is generally agreed to be a period between 10 years old and 24 years old. In many societies, however, adolescence is narrowly equated with puberty and the cycle of physical changes culminating in reproductive maturity. Adolescence has been shown to be a period where individuals gain an increasingly more stable identity status, form stable cultural orientations, and establish more salient and intimate relations with peers and romantic partners. Of all aspects of adolescent mental health, and its many influences, it is important to look at the way an Adolescent may respond to these changes. The available influencing factors such as accessibility to the internet, sexting and peer pressure. The time of adolescence is a time for the maturation and the development of the adolescents' personality, emotions and cognitive function and not just the development of the body. Maturation and the development of personality have been condensed to 5 personality traits that influence development of the maturing adolescent personality. They are:

1. Openness
2. Agreeableness
3. Emotional Stability
4. Extraversion
5. Conscientiousness.

Openness is otherwise known as intellect which includes having many interests, being imaginative and insightful. Agreeableness can be describes as being sympathetic and kind. Emotional stability is the ability to manage emotions like anxiety and the rapid changes in mood. Extraversion is being talkative, energetic and assertive. Conscientiousness includes being organized and being able to plan.

It is very important to understand these personality traits in order to understand how they influence development and maturation. As well as how they play a role in the maturation of the female adolescent. Research completed in Sweden demonstrates that maturation in personality development correlates with the mean level of agreeableness and emotional stability which were found to be increased during the adolescent period. Surprisingly there was mixed evidence of increased extraversion and openness found in the developing adolescents. An important factor that was noticed by the authors of the research was that there was a gender difference in the timing of adolescent personality maturation, as females were found to mature faster than males, even though males later catch up. Results further indicated that interindividual differences and personality profiles stabilize at an earlier age in female. These changes in physical, emotional and cognitive development brings with it changes in personality traits. The changes in personality traits can be influenced by peer pressure which over the past decade, in the literature has increasingly focused on the distinctions, such as various potential sources of peer influence on adolescent behavior and the level of influence they have. For instance, the influence of a best friend can differ from that a popular peer, role models or a larger peer networks.

CYBERBULLYING AND THE INTERNET

Childhood bullying in not only occurring in school, but has become an electronic phenomenon. With the increasing use of technology and electronic forms of communication, cyberbullying has become an increasing epidemic. The evolution of the cellphone and Wifi internet being readily available has created an increased risk for cyber bullying through texting, exposure of unwanted photograph/videos of victim, and its overuse. In the U.S., roughly 95% of teenagers report having a smartphone, cellphone or having access to one. The cellphone serves as an expeditious means of victimizing others. Cyberbully is defined as an "aggressive, intentional act carried out by a group or individual using electronic technologies of contact, repeatedly and overtime, against a victim who cannot easily defend him or herself." The bully and the victim are of unequal power. Existing research displays this form of bullying is common.

On average the rate of being either a victim of cyberbullying or a perpetrator of cyberbullying fall between the ranges of 20% to 40% nationwide. Defining features of cyberbullying include expanse of the potential audience and anonymity of the perpetrator; making this type of bullying more complex. At times the perpetrator may be unaware of the consequences of his or her actions. In recent population based studies, traditional bullying remained prevalent with girl and boys, 31.5% and 33.8% respectively. An association was observed whereby girls who are traditionally victimized tended to be both cyberbullies and cyber victims at 39.6% prevalence. This trend is more prevalent in females as compared to boys who fall at 31.7%. Of the female cyber victims 23.0% were victimized through instant messaging services and 10.3% were victimized through text messages. Of those victimized 1 in 4 people reported fear for their safety; this may indicate possible trauma associated with these events. The fear of safety is more prevalent in cyberbullying as opposed to traditional bullying. Few gender differences were further observed.

Being a cyberbully is associated with conduct issues, tobacco smoking, alcohol use, and low prosocial behaviors. On the other hand, cyber victims are more likely to experience depressive symptoms and psychosomatic symptoms including sleep disturbances, enuresis, stomach aches and headaches. Although much cyberbullying occurs outside of school, youths report affects in school. Many victim do report being fearful of going to school; this in turn escalates to severe avoidance which may lead to truancy. Involvement in cyberbullying has been shown to negatively predict perceived peer acceptance and learning in school. These symptoms should alert clinicians to be mindful of traditional and cyber bullying.

SEXTING IN ADOLESCENCE

Another aspect of adolescent mental health and increasing technology is the concept of 'Sexting.' This is defined as "sending of sexually explicit text messages or images via the internet or mobile device." In research this practice has been found to be a common behavior among adolescent. Furthermore, research has shown about 27.6% of adolescents have participating in sexting behavior. Sexting behavior can be further divided into sending, requesting, being asked for a 'sext,' or receiving a 'sext' without permission. Sexting can predict digital dating violence and is seen as an extension of offline physical harassment (touching or groping without consent). Specifically female adolescents are repeatedly requested, pressured, or coerced by other to send sexually explicit material. Often times, teenage girls partake in this behavior for fear of losing their romantic partner or preoccupied with negative social consequences. In a longitudinal cohort of female adolescents in Texas found that offline sexual coercion is associated with increased sexting behaviors. There is also a strong correlation of sexting with actual sexual behaviors, the average age was 19.02. Of those females' adolescents who experienced offline forms of sexual coercion, were more likely to participate is 'sexting' by sending, asking for, or receiving naked images without giving consent. This also remains an important public health issue as sexting is associated with increased risk of substance use, risky sexual behavior, cyber bullying, as well as reputational damage.

Sexual Behavior in Adolescence

The increase in sexting also reflects an increase in sexual behavior. According to the most recent report from the Center for Disease Control, more than half of U.S. teenagers have had their first sexual encounter by the age of 18. The mean age of first sexual intercourse was 17.3 years old for females and 17.0 years old for males. Of the teenaged females, 74% had their first sexual experience with a long term relationship and just 2% with someone they "just met." Known psychosocial risk factors for adolescent sexual intercourse include alcohol use, delinquency, and issues in school. With regards to female adolescents, early sexual activity was correlated to depressive symptoms and may also result in increased risk for unplanned pregnancy and sexually transmitted infections. Early female sexual intercourse has been associated with behavioral issues of anger and antisocial behavior. Early sexual maturity is directly related to early sexual activity. Advanced physical maturity has been linked to increase risk of risky-sexual behavior, alcohol, and substance use. An interesting point to consider is that sexual minority females including bisexual and lesbian female may be less likely to receive preventative advice leading to an increased risk of teenage pregnancies. This remains an important public health concern and points to increase sex education in school taking into account sexual orientation.

Intimate Dating Violence in Adolescence

Intimate dating violence has been associated with increased risk of sexual behavior, suicidality, and substance use. More than 1.5 million women are physically and sexually abused by an intimate partner each year. Approximately 25% of all women have experienced intimate partner violence (IPV), and approximately 25% of adolescents have experienced physical and/or sexual dating violence. Young age remains a consistent risk factor for IPV. Rate of violence against women exceeds that of males at 3 to 6 times more. Females are also 10 times more likely to be killed. Dating violence is a growing public health issue that is not adequately addressed in schools, as there are so few studies which touch upon youth and adolescent experiences.

According to one study, 1 in 5 female students from 9th to 12th grade expressed being physically or sexually abused by a dating partner after administration of a Youth Risk Survey. Most adolescent female whom experienced a form of sexual abuse also experienced physical abuse; inversely those whom had suffered physical abuse did not necessarily experience sexual abuse. Dating violence has been shown to increase the risk of sexual risky behaviors including first intercourse prior to the age of 15 and/or having 3 or more sexual partners. Studies have shown that intimate dating violence among adolescent may actually be higher than adult populations, as they are at higher risk to begin with. Younger aged adolescents are least at risk possibly due to the lower rate of dating and/or sexual activity. With an increase risk of risky sexual behaviors, there comes an increased prevalence of pregnancy at a rate of 4-6 times more likely than non-abused peers. The likelihood of contracting Human Immunodeficiency Virus (HIV) and other sexually transmitted infections also becomes prevalent.

Increased risk of eating disorder has been found to be associated with intimate dating violence. Studies have shown unhealthy weight control has been linked to dating violence and young adolescent females. Weight control methods included laxative use and vomiting with the intention of losing weight. Another concern is that adolescent females who were either physically abused or sexually abused were also more likely to have had recent suicidal ideation or suicidal attempt. This overwhelming number is at a rate of 6 to 9 times more likely to have risk for suicidality. It has been observed that the pain and humiliation of the event plays a large role in this type of suicidal behavior and in turn point to possible trauma.

Time and time again, adolescents who experience intimate dating violence are more likely to be missed and may not be connected to psychiatric treatment services. As a result, special attention must be made to symptomatology being discussed. Adolescent females which are victims of intimate dating violence had increased risk for substance use issues, namely alcohol by binge-drinking, tobacco, and cocaine abuse. It is still unclear whether substance use leads to vulnerability to dating violence or vice versa. What remains clear-cut is that dating violence and cyberbullying can lead to substance use problems.

SUBSTANCE ABUSE IN ADOLESCENCE

The results of research study has provided a better understanding of the association between peer pressure and the adoption of behaviors such as substance use and age of first sexual experience. Another study analysis was designed to assess the extent to which a teen's future levels of substance use could be predicted, and as expected, a significant effect of peer use at age 15 increased the chances of future teen substance in the following years. A study was done in Sweden on adolescents and the results exposed a robust positive association between online social network chatting and alcohol use. The study also found that online social network chatting accounted for one-fifth of the association between the peer status pathway and alcohol use. Preclinical studies have consistently shown altered sensitivity to drugs as a result of social isolation. The social environment of an individual has a profound, but complex, influence on drug use. One other significant study showed how social play behavior is highly rewarding in laboratory animals. In humans, antisocial personality traits, most prominently in the form of conduct disorder, are a prominent risk factor for drug addiction. The risks the maturing female adolescent is exposed to as a result of peer pressure are: early sexual experience, and drug use. This has a long lasting consequences on their growth, development and overall life with at least one study suggesting that chronic marijuana use, particularly when use begins in adolescence, leads to later declines in general intellectual function. Similar studies have been done showing negative outcomes are particularly salient in the contexts of earlier use onset (<age 16 years) as well as heavier and more frequent use, most often studied in relation to alcohol use. Research carried out on rats

using quinpirole which produces significant THC-like effect in the brain decreases dopamine fiber and receptor density in prefrontal cortex, and inhibits normal adult maturation of contingency degradation behavior. This is the causal relationship between actions and their consequences. Thus, rapidly maturing dopamine systems may be especially sensitive to disruption by environmental influences during adolescence, with long-term consequences on behavior and associated psychopathologies such as drug use or schizophrenia.

Table 1. Summary of adolescents and mental health

Personality Development	• Condensed to 5 personality traits that influence development of the maturing adolescent personality which include Openness, Agreeableness, Emotional Stability, Extraversion, and Conscientiousness.
Cyberbullying	• The rate of being either a victim of cyberbullying or a perpetrator of · It falls between the ranges of 5 to 20% nationwide. • Of female cyber victims 23.0% were victimized through instant messaging services and 10.3% were victimized through text messages. • Of those victimized 1 in 4 people reported fear for their safety; this may indicate possible trauma associated with these events. • Being a cyberbully is associated with conduct issues, smoking, alcohol abuse, and low prosocial behaviors.
Sexuality	• Known psychosocial risk factors for adolescent sexual intercourse include alcohol use, delinquency, and issues in school.
Intimate Dating Violence	• It is know that 25% of all women will with have experienced intimate partner violence, and approximately 25% of adolescents have experienced physical and/or sexual dating violence. • Young age remains a consistent risk factor for IPV. Rate of violence against women exceeds that of males at 3 to 6 times more. Females are also 10 times more likely to be killed. • Intimate dating violence has been associated with increased risk of sexual behavior, suicidality, and substance abuse.
Substance Abuse	• There is a positive association between peer pressure and the adoption of behaviors such as substance use and age of first sexual experience. • Substance use during the adolescent years predicts future use of substances in later years.

References

Allen JP, Chango J, Szwedo D, Schad M, Marston E. Predictors of susceptibility to peer influence regarding substance use in adolescence. *Child Dev*. 2011;83(1):33750. https://www.ncbi.nlm.nih.gov/pmc/articles/PMC3390749/.

Baldry, Anna Costanza, Anna Sorrentino, David P. Farrington. *Cyberbullying and Cyber victimization versus parental supervision, monitoring and control of adolescents' online activities*. https://doi.org/10.1016/J.CHILDYOUTH.2018.11.058.

Betts, Lucy. Karin Spenser, and Sarah Gardener. "Adolescents' Involvement in Cyber Bullying and Perceptions of School: The Importance of Perceived Peer Acceptance for Female Adolescents." *Sex Roles*, March 2017, 471.

HyeJeong Choie, PhD, Joris Van Outsel, MSc, and Jeff Temple, PhD., "Association between Sexting and Sexual Coercion among Female Adolescents." *J Adolesc,* December 2016, 164-68. Accessed December 28, 2018. https://www.ncbi.nlm.nih.gov/pmc/articles/PMC5127271/.

John, O. P., Naumann, L. P., & Soto, C. J. (2008). Paradigm Shift to the Integrative Big-Five Trait Taxonomy: History, Measurement, and Conceptual Issues. In O. P. John, R. W. Robins, & L. A. Pervin (Eds.), *Handbook of personality: Theory and research* (pp. 114-158). New York, NY: Guilford Press. https://pages.uoregon.edu/sanjay/bigfive.html.

Klimstra, Theo A. William W. Hale III, Quinten A. W. Raaijmakers, Susan J. T. Branje, and Wim H. J. Meeus, *Research Centre Adolescent Development*, Utrecht University, Utrecht, The Netherlands. https://www.researchgate.net/publication/24222404_Maturation_of_Personality_in_Adolescence.

Mahalik, James R., McPherran, Caitlin, Lombardi, Jacqueline, Sims, Rebekah, Levine, Coley, Alicia, Doyle, Lynch. *Gender, male-typicality, and social norms predicting adolescent alcohol intoxication and marijuana use.* DOI link: https://doi.org/10.1016/J.SOCSCIMED.2015.08.013. Published: 2015-10.

Pringle, Jan Katherine Mills, and John McAteer. "The Physiology of Adolescent Sexual Behavior: A Systematic Review." *Cogent Social Sciences 3* (August 15, 2017): 10-14. https://www.ncbi.nlm.nih.gov/pmc/articles/PMC5692360/pdf/oass-3-1368858.pdf.

Sansone, Randy, MD. "Cell Phones: The Psychosocial Risks." *Innovations in Clinical Neuroscience* 10, no. 1, 33-35. Accessed December 28, 2018. https://www.ncbi.nlm.nih.gov/pmc/articles/PMC3579483/pdf/icns_10_1_33.pdf.

Silverman, Jay, PhD, Anita Raj, PhD, Lorelei Mucci, MPH, and Jeanne Hathaway, MPH. "Dating Violence Against Adolescent Girls And Associated Substance Use, Unhealthy, Weight Control, Sexual Risk Behavior, Pregnancy, and Suicidality." *JAMA Psychiatry.* 286, no. 5, 572-79. Accessed December 28, 2018. file:///C:/Users/mbadillo/Downloads/joc02015(1).pdf.

Sourander, Andre, MD, PhD, Klomek Anat, PhD, and Ikonen, Maria, MA., "Psychosocial Risk Factors Associated with Cyberbullying Among Adolescents." *Arch Gen Psychiatry.* 67, no. 7 (July 2010): 720-27. Accessed January 4, 2019. https://jamanetwork.com/journals/jamapsychiatry/.

Trezza, V., Baarendse, P. J. J. & Vanderschuren, L. J. M. J. *Psychopharmacology* (2014) 231: 1715. https://doi.org/10.1007/s00213-014-3471-z.

In: Women's Pearls
Editors: S. Fink and P. Korenis

ISBN: 978-1-53616-103-8

Chapter 3

PREMENSTRUAL DYSPHORIC DISORDER IN HISTORY

Maria T. Carvajal, MD, Maliha Desmukh, MD and Ashaki Martin, MD*

Bronx-Care Hospital,
Icahn School of Medicine at Mount Sinai, New York, NY, US

ABSTRACT

Descriptions of premenstrual dysphoria and physical symptoms date back to the time of Hippocrates when a woman's monthly menstrual cycle was proclaimed to "purge her bad humors". Trotula of Salerno, an 11th century female gynecologist noted in "The Diseases of Women" "there are young women who are relieved when the menses are called forth".

In 1931 Dr. Robert Frank, through his case series, discussed women who experienced tension with a variety of emotional symptoms and worsening of their concurrent medical conditions during the few days prior to menstruation. In 1952 the Diagnostic and Statistical Manual of Mental Disorders, 3rd edition (DSM III-R) laid out the initial diagnostic criteria for "Late luteal phase dysphoric disorder" in Appendix A

* Corresponding Author's E-mail: AMartin@bronxleb.org.

emphasizing the timing and severity of symptoms by designating a minimum of five symptoms with predictable onset and offset in the late luteal and early follicular phases of the menstrual cycle. In Diagnostic and Statistical Manual of Mental Disorders 4th edition (DSM – IV) the term "Premenstrual Dysphoric Disorder" emerged replacing "late luteal phase dysphoric disorder" and brought with it a diagnostic criterion that was slightly modified. However, it remained in the Appendix category as the work group believed more research was required to confirm the distinctiveness of the category from other mood disorders, and to identify its true prevalence and specific criteria.

The Mood Disorder Work Group for Diagnostic and Statistical Manual of Mental Disorders, 5th edition (DSM -5), consisting of a panel of international experts in women's mental health, the task force was assigned to extensively review research to evaluate previous criteria for Premenstrual dysphoric disorder (PMDD), to ascertain whether enough support existed to include it as a separate diagnostic category. The review was to verify if any changes were needed to be made to the existing diagnostic criteria, in light of new research in the field. The result was the shift from Appendix A to a separate diagnosis within the Mood Disorders section in 2013.

The benefit of including PMDD as a full-fledged diagnosis allows for more research focusing on its pathophysiology as well as the Food and Drug Administration approving several pharmacological agents. This category also describes a group of individuals who are otherwise not represented by other psychiatric diagnostic criteria's. Furthermore, multiple studies report that women with PMDD who experience significant functional impairment in various aspects of their lives, demonstrate improvement when in treatment.

Some believed that a diagnostic category focusing on the female's menstrual cycle would "pathologize" reproductive functioning in women and would lead to the insinuation that women may not be able to carry out tasks during the premenstrual phase of the cycle. However, being that PMDD is prevalent in a small minority of women, this leaves the generalization of such statements and inferences of disability in all women grossly inapplicable.

Introduction

Women somatopsychic illness has been found to be directly related to the hormonal changes that occur during the menstrual cycle. Current literature provides detailed explanation regarding the effect of changes in sex steroid levels and its influence on changes in mood, based on the phase of the ovulatory cycle. These changes or imbalances occur during the menstrual cycle, from menarche to menopause, on a monthly basis. Premenstrual syndrome (PMS) is defined by affective symptoms (depression, angry outbursts), and physical symptoms (breast pain, bloating). PMDD is a severe form of PMS, which is defined by the presence of five symptoms, in the week before menses and end by the post menses week. In premenstrual dysphoric disorder (PMDD), symptoms of anger, irritability, and internal tension are prominent.

Premenstrual dysphoric syndrome has been described in the Diagnostic and statistical Manual of Mental Disorders, fifth edition (DSM-V), under the depressive disorder's category. In this chapter we aim to provide a review of the presentation, diagnosis and treatment of one of the most common psychiatric illness related to hormonal changes in women. A thorough history, which gathers the necessary information pertaining to the evolution of symptoms and its correlation to the different phases of the menstrual cycle, is important in determining the diagnosis.

EPIDEMIOLOGY

Premenstrual dysphoric disorder (PMDD), can be differentiated from premenstrual syndrome (PMS) when DSM-V criteria is strictly applied. PMDD requires at least five symptoms, including one affective symptom, such as mood swings, irritability, and/or depression. The prevalence of PMS and PMDD in the population has been overestimated due to the lack of strict diagnostic criteria. It is estimated that PMS affects three to eight percent of women, and PMDD truly affects two percent of women. A study by Yonkers et al., showed that black women were less likely to experience PMDD than white women. The prevalence of PMDD was 2.9 percent among black women compared to 4.4 percent among white women.

PREMENSTRUAL SYNDROME

PMS is cyclic and recurrent and requires at least three consecutive months, of physical, emotional, behavioral, and cognitive symptoms. The characteristics of the syndrome are based on the timeline and correlation of symptoms with the menstrual cycle phases. The symptoms start during the luteal phase of the menstrual cycle and resolves shortly after the start of the menses. A study conducted by Freeman et al., of 1081 women who requested PMS treatment at an academic medical center, analyzed a prospective daily symptom ratings and functional impairment data. In the study, six core symptoms were identified that included anxiety/tension, mood swings, aches, appetite/food cravings, cramps, and decreased interest in activities

PREMENSTRUAL DYSPHORIC DISORDER

Premenstrual dysphoric disorder (PMDD) is a psychosomatic illness, where affective symptoms such as mood swings, irritability, anger, increased interpersonal conflicts, depressed mood, anxiety, tension, lack of interest, difficulty in concentration, lethargy, lack of energy, changes in appetite, hypersomnia or insomnia, aches in breasts, joints or muscles, edema, weight gain, paresthesia, syncope, and bloating sensations are present. At least five of the aforementioned symptoms need to be present in the week prior to menses. The symptoms start to improve after menses, and they are resolved by the postmenses week.

MENSTRUAL CYCLE

The menstrual cycle is classified into two phases; the follicular phase and the luteal phase. The follicular phase extends from the first day of menses until ovulation and estrogen levels increase during this phase.

Gonadotrophin releasing hormones are then secreted, followed by a surge in luteinizing hormone (LH) and follicle stimulating hormone (FSH) and a fall in the estrogen levels. Ovulation occurs about twelve hours following the peak of the luteinizing hormone (LH) surge. Following ovulation, the luteal phase ensues, which is marked by peak serum levels of estrogen and progesterone; this then culminates in menstruation if pregnancy does not occur.

DIAGNOSIS

Menstrual cycles history should be obtained in a detailed manner, to asses the initiation and evolution of symptoms surrounding and during the menstrual cycle. Prospective data of at least two months should be obtained. Symptoms may be recorded with the Daily Record of Severity of Problems (DRSP) form. PMS diagnosis is made, if there is one to four symptoms present, which may be physical, behavioral, or affective or five or more physical or behavioral symptoms. For PMDD diagnosis, there should be five or more symptoms present, with one of them being an affective symptom. DSM-V criteria should be followed in order to confirm the diagnosis.

Hormonal levels, Thyroid-Stimulating Hormone (TSH), Human Chorionic Gonadotropin Hormone (hCG) and Follicle-Stimulating Hormone (FSH), should be obtained in women with irregular menstrual cycles, but is not indicated if the irregularity is related to menopause. Hormonal levels are obtained to rule out diseases that can present with similar symptomatology, such as mood disorders, depression, and secondary causes of amenorrhea.

The course of psychiatric illness is directly influenced by menstrual cycle patterns. In Premenstrual dysphoric disorder (PMDD), depressed mood, mood lability, irritability and increased interpersonal conflicts are confined to the luteal phase when estrogen levels have declined, which is followed by an asymptomatic period after the onset menses. Inoue et al. (2007), in their study which compared serotonergic function in

Premenstrual dysphoric disorder (PMDD) subjects versus normal controls using neuroendocrine challenge tests found higher serotonergic function in the follicular phase, while the luteal phase was characterized by lower serotonergic function.

Hormonal fluctuation plays a key role in the pathogenesis of Premenstrual dysphoric disorder (PMDD). Research has shown that women with Premenstrual dysphoric disorder (PMDD) have normal ovarian hormonal levels, however, they exhibit an altered sensitivity to the fluctuations in hormone levels. Estrogen affects regulation of mood and behavior by altering expression of the of the Serotonin receptor (5HT2A receptor) and serotonin transporter (SERT) genes. Low estrogen levels were linked to decreased expression of the SERT gene. Women with Premenstrual syndrome (PMS) and Premenstrual dysphoric disorder (PMDD) display abnormalities in serotonin particularly in the luteal phase when there is a drop in the estrogen levels. Progesterone and its metabolite allopregnolone are also important in the etiology of Premenstrual dysphoric disorder (PMDD). There is a rise in these hormones during the luteal phase, with a rapid decline around menses; it is hypothesized that this chronic exposure to progesterone and subsequent withdrawal may be a causal factor in the development of Premenstrual dysphoric disorder (PMDD). Animal models which demonstrate that progesterone withdrawal in rats were associated with Premenstrual dysphoric disorder (PMDD) symptoms such as social withdrawal and anhedonia support this hypothesis.

TREATMENT

Selective Serotonin Reuptake Inhibitors (SSRIs)

PMDD is a chronic cyclical disorder in which serotoninergic function is reduced during the luteal phase. Several treatment modalities have been proven to be beneficial in PMDD and severe PMS, but the selective serotonin reuptake inhibitors (SSRIs) have emerged as first-line therapy.

The SSRIs can be administered continuously throughout the entire month, intermittently from ovulation to the onset of menstruation, or semi-intermittently with dosage increases during the late luteal phase. The treatment of choice is a SSRI; either sertraline or modified-release paroxetine. The American Psychiatric Association (APA) has listed SSRI as approved medication to treat this disorder and they recommend that treatment be administered throughout the menstrual cycle. Treatment regimen should be chosen based on a physician's assessment of onset and duration of symptoms, and the patient's preference. Women with low level of symptoms should receive treatment during the menstrual cycle on a daily basis. If irregular menstrual cycles or failed intermittent treatment occurs, continuous treatment should be considered. When symptoms appear more during the week before menses, treatment during the luteal phase might be beneficial. Women who can identify the onset of symptoms for a specific period might benefit from therapy that starts at the onset of symptoms

The following are the most frequently used SSRIs in the treatment of PMDD; Fluoxetine in doses of 20-60 milligrams per day, with a maximum dose of 80 mg per day; Paroxetine 12.5 to 30 milligrams per day, to be administered in the morning; and Sertraline 50 to 200 milligrams per day, in the morning. Sertraline should be up titrated by 50 mg/day at each menstrual cycle or 100 mg/day if taken during the luteal phase only. Other SSRIs that may be used include: Citalopram 20 to 30 mg/day and Escitalopram 10 to 20 mg/day.

The benefits of treatment are noticed within one to two weeks of initiation. Improvement in mood and physical symptoms has been reported to be about 50 to 60% during this period. Long term treatment efficacy has not been proven, but specialists have recommended continuation of treatment until menopause has occurred, as there is evidence that supports the recurrence of symptoms when treatment is stopped.

Second Line Therapies

Oral Contraceptives

The Food and Drug Administration (FDA) has approved hormonal treatment with Drospirenone and ethinyl estradiol for PMDD treatment in women who choose to use an oral contraceptive method. The starting dose is a 3 mg drospirenone/20 mcg ethinyl estradiol oral contraceptive (OC), with a four-day pill-free interval; if PMDD symptoms persist or if there is breakthrough bleeding that does not resolve, the dose can be increased to a 3 mg drospirenone/30 mcg ethinyl estradiol combination. If symptoms continue despite a higher estrogen dose, a trial of continuous hormonal oral contraceptive should be used. Continuous therapy with levonorgestrel (90 mcg) and ethinyl estradiol (20 mcg) may be an option. When choosing a prolonged OC treatment, a detailed medical history and evaluation of the individual's risk of venous thromboembolism should be considered, since Drospirenone has higher risk of venous thromboembolism when compared to Levonorgestrel and other progestins.

GnRH Agonist

Gonadotropin releasing hormone (GnRH) analogues are used in cases where intolerance or failed treatment with SSRIs or OCPs has been reported. The associated risk of osteoporosis when GnRH agonists are used for a 6 month period, has limited its use. GnRH agonists can be administered simultaneously with estrogen and progestin to avoid menopausal symptoms and bone loss.

Nonpharmacological Therapies

These include lifestyle modifications which may include, aerobic exercise, consumption of complex carbohydrates and frequent meals, relaxation training, light therapy, acupuncture and cognitive behavioral therapy. Limited data exists on the efficacy of these interventions.

Table 1. History, diagnostic criteria, and treatments of PMDD

- DSM III-R was the first time mood symptoms preceding menstruation was mentioned in Appendix A section under Late luteal phase dysphoric disorder with an initial diagnostic criteria
- DSM IV slightly modified this diagnostic criteria and renamed the Late luteal phase dysphoric disorder as premenstrual dysphoric disorder, but continued to classify it within the Appendix A category
- The Mood Disorder work group for DSM -5 reviewed literature citing statistical prevalence, degree of disability of those suffering from PMDD, and response to treatments, and came to the conclusion that PMDD warranted being included as a separate diagnostic category within the Mood Disorders section
- The symptoms of Premenstrual Dysphoric Disorder (PMDD) are prominent in the luteal phase of the menstrual cycle.
- Low estrogen levels which are characteristic of the luteal phase are related to decreased serotonergic gene expression and overall decline in serotonergic function
- The first line treatment for Premenstrual Dysphoric Disorder (PMDD) is selective serotonin reuptake inhibitors (SSRIs)
- Second line treatment for Premenstrual Dysphoric Disorder (PMDD) is oral contraceptive
- Nonpharmacological treatments for Premenstrual Dysphoric Disorder (PMDD) include aerobic exercise, relaxation training, light therapy, acupuncture and cognitive behavioral therapy.

References

Freeman EW, Halberstadt SM, Rickels K, Legler JM, Lin H, Sammel MD. (2011) Core symptoms that discriminate premenstrual syndrome. *J Womens Health* (Larchmt) Jan; 20(1):29-35. Epub 2010.

Frank RT. (1931) The hormonal causes of premenstrual tension. *Arch Neurol Psychiatry*, 26, pp. 1053-1057.

Lieberman Jeffrey, Allan Tasman. (2006) *Handbook of Psychiatric drugs*. John Wiley & Sons Ltd, (West Sussex, England).

Mason-Hohl E. (1940) *The Diseases of Women, by Trotula of Salerno: A Translation of Passionibus Mulierum Curandorum* by Elizabeth Mason-Hohl, MD. Los Angeles: Ward Ritchie Press.

Pearlstein T, Halbreich U, Batzar E, Brown C, Endicott J, Frank E, Freeman EW, Harrison WM, Haskett RF, Stout AL, Yonkers KA. Psychosocial functioning in women with premenstrual dysphoric disorder before and after treatment with sertraline or placebo. *J Clin Psychiatry*, 2000;61:101–109.

Rapkin AJ, Lewis EI. (2013) Treatment of premenstrual dysphoric disorder. *Womens Health* (Lond). PubMed.

Sadock BJ, Sadock VA, Ruiz P. (2015) *Synopsis of Psychiatry, Eleventh Edition.* (Philadelphia: Wolters Kluwer.

Shah NR, Jones JB, Aperi J, Shemtov R, Karne A, Borenstein J. (2008) *Selective serotonin reuptake inhibitors for premenstrual syndrome and premenstrual dysphoric disorder: A meta-analysis*. Obstet Gynecol.

Steiner M, et al. Fluoxetine improves functional work capacity in women with premenstrual dysphoric disorder. *Arch Womens Ment Health.* 2003;6:71–77.

Steiner M, et al. (2006) Expert guidelines for the treatment of severe PMS, PMDD, and comorbidities: The role of SSRIs. *J Womens Health* (Larchmt).

Yonkers Kimberly et al., *Epidemiology and pathogenesis of premenstrual syndrome and premenstrual dysphoric disorder.* Edited by Robert L Barbieri, MD, William F Crowley, Jr, MD Deputy Kathryn A Martin, MD: UpToDate 2018.

In: Women's Pearls
Editors: S. Fink and P. Korenis
ISBN: 978-1-53616-103-8

Chapter 4

The Impact of Infertility on Mental Health

Panagiota Korenis, MD
Bronx-Care Health System,
Icahn School of Medicine at Mount Sinai, New York, NY, US;
Albert Einstein College of Medicine, New York, NY, US

Introduction

The road to parenthood while joyous and magical for some can also be wrought with complications and uncertainty for others. Despite advancements in medical knowledge, clinicians are still not able to predict how a woman's journey to motherhood will transpire. Infertility is defined as an inability to get pregnant after one year (twelve months) of trying to become pregnant. Couples of reproductive age across all cultures and societies experience infertility with a prevalence of 10-15%. Currently, couples presenting with infertility has increased and this is thought to be due to a variety of factors including: postponement of wanting to have children, innovative and successful techniques for infertility treatment, and increasing awareness of options available for a couple who has infertility. Not only have these innovative technologies inspired couples to pursue having children when they thought there were no options, this has also shed light on the psychological impact of infertility. Studies have also begun to study psychiatric illness and infertility as well as the impact of prolonged infertility and invasive infertility treatments on women's wellbeing.

Psychological Impact of Infertility

Becoming a mother is one of the major transitions in adult life for women. The impact of not being able to become pregnant presents as an isolating, shameful experience for a woman and it is not uncommon that there may be an impact on her mood. Symptoms including: anger, depression, anxiety, changes in the marital dynamic, sexual dysfunction, and social isolation are just some of the potential consequences of infertility. Couples may experience stigma, a sense of loss, and diminished self-esteem during the period of infertility. In general, when a couple is faced with infertility, the level of distress is higher in the female partner than in the male. It is important to note however, that when infertility is attributed to the male partner, men's distress rate is similar to women.

Commonly, depression, anxiety and stress are considered consequences of infertility. A growing number of studies show that depression is significantly higher in infertile couples than in fertile controls. Stress, depression and anxiety are described as common consequences of infertility. In infertile couples, anxiety has also been shown to be higher than in the general population. Understanding the role of psychiatric illness in the development of infertility remains a debate. No studies have been able to confirm that those with a history of mental illness are more likely to become infertile.

Proposed theories whereby depression may directly result in infertility involves an elevated prolactin level during the depressed state, disruption of the hypothalamic-pituitary-adrenal axis (HPPA), and dysregulated thyroid hormone (in particular, subclinical hypothyroidism). One study suggests that depression is associated with abnormal regulation of the hormone that regulated ovulation, the luteinizing hormone. Changes in immune function associated with stress may also adversely affect reproductive function. Further studies are needed to better understand the impact of depression on reproductive success. Another theory proposes the notion that cumulative stress may also be associated with infertility and increase the risk for comorbid anxiety and depression.

INFERTILITY TREATMENT

Reproductive failure, on its own may cause high levels of emotional dysregulation infertility treatment itself is also associated with increased anxiety and depression. Evidence suggests that for women undergoing in vitro fertilization (IVF) they are more likely to be depressed, less confident and had a lower self esteem when compared to fertile women. For women who have experienced failed IVF treatments, the results are more dire and the impact on a women's mental health and wellbeing that much more severe. Current literature also proposes that women who undergo multiple failed trials are at further risk for developing depressive symptoms.

Studies have also assessed the outcome of infertility treatment and noted that success may be influenced by emotional health. Mood state and stress are considered common predictors of outcome in assisted reproduction. Many studies have concluded that being distressed while pursuing infertility treatment directly results in lower pregnancy rates in women.

What Can Be Done to Combat Emotional Dysfunction during Infertility?

It is well known that psychological symptoms interfere with fertility. Given this, there has been a lot of interest to combat the impact of depression and anxiety throughout infertility treatment. Studies have focused on identifying treatment options to ensure optimal success of infertility treatment, the ability to continue ongoing treatment if necessary.

Cognitive behavioral group psychotherapy and support groups have been well researched and noted to decrease mood symptoms, as well as increase the rate of fertility. In a year-long follow-up study, Domar and colleagues compared rates of conception of women undergoing fertility treatment who were randomized to a group cognitive behavioral therapy (CBT) designed to lower mood and anxiety symptoms to no group treatment. Pregnancy rates were significantly increased for the women who participated in CBT treatment and group therapy. Other studies have assessed the impact of couples counseling aimed at decreasing depression and anxiety and pregnancy outcomes. Patients who participated in these counseling sessions showed significantly more pregnancies than their counterparts who did not.

While no studies have assessed the potential impact of psychodynamic psychotherapy, dialectical behavioral therapy or other formal psychotherapeutic modality, it is posited that any psychotherapeutic intervention aimed at ameliorating mood symptoms and decreasing stress levels would be helpful for these women.

There is little research around psychopharmacological treatment of women who struggle with infertility. It is important to note that this population is at risk of experiencing symptoms consistent with major depressive disorder, anxiety disorders, sleep disturbances that may warrant pharmacological intervention. Despite this reality, many women who are experiencing infertility with comorbid depression or anxiety may avoid medications that could impact their pregnancy. There are no studies that suggest that antidepressants or anxiolytic medications, medications commonly prescribed for major depression or anxiety disorders negatively impact fertility. Additionally, current studies suggest that there are some medications which can be safely administered during pregnancy.

Infertility and the Couple

Men and women each account for 35-40% of infertility rates while the remainder of cases are attributed to unknown causes. The majority of the literature focuses on the impact of infertility on women, however, a growing body of evidence does suggest that there is an impact on men as well. Traditional notions of masculinity, like traditional notions of femininity revolve around the biological ability to bare children. The inability to fulfill this biological role leads to feelings of shame and humiliation. This sense of shame and humiliation may lead to isolation, resentment and can negatively impact the relationship. Prolonged infertility can have devastating effects on a relationship. During fertility treatment, intimacy may be compromised as love making becomes regimented, less spontaneous and can lead to performance anxiety for both men and women.

Understanding that there can be a negative impact of infertility on men as well as women should encourage couples to seek psychotherapeutic interventions like couples counseling as early as possible. Openly discussing the challenges of infertility as a couple has been shown to prevent isolation and shame.

The stress of both infertility and fertility treatment can potentiate existing problems, such financial issues and poor communication. It can also lead to the development of new problems. Additionally, couples may be challenged with how far and how much they will "work" to conceive a child. These new stressors may also happen when women are taking hormones that impact mood and anxiety symptoms.

While disparities in healthcare are not unique, it is important to note that for couples who struggle with infertility, psychosocial stressors have been shown to lead to worse outcomes for this population. Fertility treatments may not be covered by insurance or even if they are, the hormone therapy may have costly co-pays. Additionally, infertility treatment involves frequent medical visits that require consistency and transportation may not be provided by the medical clinic or patients may not have flexible work schedules to make the commitment to get to appointments.

When to Pursue Mental Health Treatment

It is normal to experience a multitude of emotions in the process of pursuing infertility treatment. However, when a woman experiences the following symptoms over a prolonged period of time, it is vital to consider reaching out to a mental health professional. Symptoms include: loss of interest, feelings of sadness, interpersonal difficulties, obsessive thoughts related to infertility, inability to complete tasks or focus, insomnia, thoughts about death or suicide, feelings of shame or humiliation and social isolation.

It is also helpful to consult with a mental health professional when a couple is exploring other options to build their family, considering surrogacy or egg donation or having difficulty communicating as a couple.

Table 1. Infertility specific mood symptoms

Infertility Specific Mood Symptoms
Strained interpersonal relationship, change in relationship dynamics
Intense anger or bitterness
Difficulty thinking about anything other than infertility
Social isolation
Feeling of worthlessness and that you are not fulfilling your biological role as a woman
Notion that every month when your menses comes you are mourning the loss of your unborn child
Intimacy with your partner is "structured", non spontaneous and following your ovulation cycle
Shame and humiliation

REFERENCES

Burns L.H. “Psychiatric Aspects of Infertility and Infertility Treatments,” *Psychiatric Clinics of North America* (Dec. 2007): Vol. 30, No. 4, pp. 689–716.

Chiaffarino, F., Baldini M., Scarduelli C., “Prevalence and incidence of depressive and anxious symptoms in couples undergoing assisted reproductive treatment in an Italian infertility department” *European Journal of Obstetrics & Gynecology and Reproductive Biology,* Volume 158, Issue 2, 2011, pp. 235-241.

Cousineau T.M., et al. “Psychological Impact of Infertility,” *Best Practice & Research: Clinical Obstetrics and Gynaecology* (April 2007): Vol. 21, No. 2, pp. 293–308.

Joja O.D., D. Dinu, D. Paun “Psychological Aspects of Male Infertility. An Overview” *Procedia - Social and Behavioral Sciences*, Volume 187, 2015, pp. 359-363.

Li Ying Ying, Lai Har Wu, Alice Yuen Loke “Gender differences in experiences with and adjustments to infertility: A literature review” *International Journal of Nursing Studies*, Volume 52, Issue 10, 2015, pp. 1640-1652.

Murugappan G., Li S., Lathi R.B., Baker V.L., Eisenberg M.L. “Increased risk of incident chronic medical conditions in infertile women: analysis of US claims data” *American Journal of Obstetrics and Gynecology,* Volume 220, 2019.

The Practice Committee of the American Society for Reproductive Medicine. “Child-Rearing Ability and the Provision of Fertility Services,” *Fertility and Sterility* (Sept. 2004): Vol. 82, Suppl. 1, pp. S208–11.

Zarbo C., Brugnera A., Compare A., Candeloro I., Secomandi R., Betto E., Fusi F., Marabini R., Malandrino C., Carnelli M., Trezzi G., Bondi E., Rabboni M., Frigerio L. “Perfectionistic traits and importance given to parenthood are associated with infertility-related quality of life in a sample of infertile women with and without endometriosis” *Sexual and Reproductive Healthcare*, Volume 17, 2018.

In: Women's Pearls
Editors: S. Fink and P. Korenis
ISBN: 978-1-53616-103-8

Chapter 5

PERINATAL MENTAL HEALTH

Viviana Chiappetta, MD* and Alejandra Cattan, MD
Bronx-Care Hospital,
Icahn School of Medicine at Mount Sinai, New York, NY, US

INTRODUCTION

Historically, pregnancy was thought to be a time of protection from psychiatric disorders, but the available research has since demonstrated that rates of mood disorders are approximately equivalent in pregnant and non-childbearing populations.

Anxiety and mood disorders are very common during the perinatal period. Help seeking is often delayed due to shame and stigma, and diagnosis is often missed due to misinterpretation of symptoms.

* Corresponding Author's Email: VChiappe@bronxleb.org.

EPIDEMIOLOGY OF ANTENATAL ANXIETY AND MAJOR DEPRESSION

The study of perinatal depression has often focused on the hypothesized role of changes in hormone concentrations during pregnancy and the postpartum period. To date, there is little evidence to support an etiology or symptomatology of depression that differs between pregnancy and other life stages, and depressive symptoms and diagnostic criteria for depressive disorders do not differ for pregnant women.

Anxiety is common during pregnancy and may be particularly pronounced when comorbid with depression. The incidence of new mental disorders and their prevalence during pregnancy seem to be similar to the 12-month incidence of mental disorders in women of the same age group without pregnancy. Major depression occurs during pregnancy with a prevalence rate between 3 and 9% (Halbreich U, et al. 2014). Pregnancy appears to increase the risk of obsessive-compulsive disorder (OCD) and anxiety disorders.

RISK FACTORS

The risk factors for depression during pregnancy are similar to those for postpartum depression. They include having a history of depression, lacking social support, having an unintended pregnancy, being of lower socioeconomic status, being exposed to domestic violence, being single, having anxiety, and having stressful life events. In addition, women with depression during pregnancy have an elevated risk of postpartum depression, which can have a significant impact on the health and well-being of both mothers and infants.

IMPACT OF DEPRESSION DURING PREGNANCY

Untreated, peripartum disorders can have especially long-term consequences, not only for the mother but also for the whole family and specially for the child. A higher rate of perinatal complications, preterm deliveries, low birth weight, postpartum depression have been reported. Recent research has shown how maternal stress, anxiety and depression can adversely influence a child's early and later development. It has been proposed that the mechanism of that is the result of the biological substrates of depression, such as activation of the HPA (hypothalamic pituitary-adrenal) axis that primes the fetus itself to depression in later life, and that activation of the maternal HPA axis leading to placenta hypersecretion of corticotropin-releasing factor with adverse effects of the fetus and on labor. However, studies showed conflictive data between anxiety and cortisol levels.

PERINATAL MATERNAL DEPRESSION

Up to 70% of pregnant women endorse depressive symptoms, with 10-16% fulfilling diagnostic criteria for MDD (Weissman, et al, 1995). In fact, over 10% of women presenting for evaluation of postpartum depression report symptom onset actually occurred during pregnancy (Riecher-Rössler, A and Meir Steiner 2005).

Studies that have looked at depression during pregnancy have shown associations with poor obstetrical outcomes including preterm delivery, postpartum depression, and neonatal symptoms. A recent study of pregnant women comparing the effects of untreated depressive symptoms, use of selective serotonin reuptake inhibitors (SSRIs), and no depressive symptoms or use of SSRIs found that untreated depressive symptoms were associated with lower total fetal body growth and head growth during pregnancy.

Depression during pregnancy has also been associated with greater developmental delays in infants in more than one study, although these studies were based on self-report of depression, another study that used more objective assessments of depression did not find an association.

In addition to concerns about the impact of depression on the fetus and neonate, there is interest in its impact on the mother's health, beyond the usual concerns related to depression, such as vegetative symptoms, self – harm, suicide, or psychosis in severe cases.

Much is less known about the impact of depression on the pregnancy, the fetus, the neonate and the mother compared with the impact of antidepressants. The lack of knowledge is particularly troubling given that the majority of women with depression do not receive treatment during pregnancy. In a study of 276 women at high risk for depression based on depression screening, only 20% were receiving any treatment for depression. Among those with a diagnosis of major depression, 33% were receiving depression treatment (Flynn, H, et al. 2006). Although women were more likely to receive treatment if they had a history of major depression before pregnancy, a history of psychiatric treatment, or greater depression severity, having a current episode of depression did not predict treatment.

LIFE TRANSITIONS

Pregnancy and puerperium are important life transitions. Women and their families undergo major changes in relationships and role expectations. Many women are faced with decisions about returning to work or staying at home with their newborn. Conflicts often arise regarding child care, parenting, or sexual intimacy during pregnancy and postpartum period. The perinatal period is an interpersonal event that is characterized by relationship changes. Perinatal depression and anxiety are associated with difficulties in resolving these interpersonal changes.

Antidepressant Use and Relapse Risk of Major Depression in Pregnancy

Among pregnant women who take antidepressants, the highest prevalence of use is during the first trimester (2%-3.7%). Rates of use during pregnancy are somewhat lower than those of women taking antidepressants before (2.9%-6.6%) and after pregnancy (7%). It seems to be a trend towards decreasing antidepressant use from the first trimester (3.7%) to the second (1.6%) to the third (1.1%) (Yonkers, KA, et al. 2011). This trend may reflect provider and patient concerns about the relationship between third trimester exposure and poor neonatal adaptation syndrome. Even when women take antidepressants during pregnancy, treatment is often inadequate, with almost 8% taking antidepressants prescribed at dosages lower than those generally recommended (Ververs, T, et al. 2006).

Many women stop taking antidepressants during pregnancy, but are not aware that research indicates that women who discontinue their medication are at much higher risk for recurrence of depression.

Relapse risk have been examined in those women who continue or cease antidepressants during pregnancy. Studies showed that women who ceased antidepressant treatment during pregnancy showed significantly higher relapse rates than those who remained on their preconception dose of medication throughout pregnancy (68% vs. 26%) (Cohen LS, et al. 2006). A study of women who abruptly discontinued antidepressants on becoming pregnant found 31% developed suicidal ideation (Einarson A, et al. 2001).

Assessment of Major Depression in Pregnancy

It is important to distinguish between women with distressing depressive symptoms and those that meet the full diagnostic criteria for a major depressive disorder. Making a diagnosis of major depressive disorder in pregnancy is complicated by the fact that there are overlapping symptoms between major depression and pregnancy-related symptoms. Studies have found that some of the typical somatic depressive disorders such as sleep, appetite, and energy level did not differ well between depressed and non-depressed pregnant women. By contrast, more cognitive symptoms of depression, such as feeling of worthless or guilty, and difficulties on concentrating, were even more remarkable. Previous history of depression should also be elicited as well as her treatment response as this will give an indication of what will be beneficial for her current episode of depression. The differential diagnosis of bipolar depression should also be considered, so asking about episodes of mania or hypomania is essential, especially when there is a family history of bipolar disorder (Galbally, M, et al. 2016).

Psychopharmacological Treatment of Depression in Pregnancy

Guidelines specific to the perinatal period suggest treatment is recommended when there has been a failure of response to psychosocial interventions or significant and debilitating symptoms of depression. There is an absence of specific evidence examining the effectiveness of antidepressant medication for depression in pregnancy. If antidepressant medication is being considered, is important to conduct a careful risk-benefit analysis.

Clinical Approach to Treating Women during Pregnancy: Risk-Benefit Analysis

The clinical approach to treating depressed pregnant women can be extremely challenging because there is no "one" correct or absolutely safe answer. However, if the clinician makes a rigorous and consistent approach to collect the information this facilitate the woman to make an informed decision.

In counseling patients with depressive illness, it is important to break down the risks and benefits of treatment options into each phase: preconception, first trimester, second trimester, third trimester and neonatal. Each phase has its own risks and benefits of treatment types for individual women, and the choices and decisions may change depending on the stage of pregnancy and the woman's symptoms and circumstances. Another important factor in counseling women is to discuss the risks both of the treatments and of untreated depression, including the data on the impact of depression on pregnancy outcomes.

For an individual woman, it is important to assess her own history of depression: the duration, recurrence, and severity of her symptoms and episodes, her history of self –harm tendencies as well as use of alcohol, drugs, and tobacco when not receiving treatment. As well as her access to different types of treatments, her social supports, the opinions about treatment of those who support her during the pregnancy (partner; mother; friend; obstetrician and pediatrician), her family history, her family situation, especially any evidence of abuse or violence, her responsibility for other children, her need for stability of mood, to be able to work and perform other tasks, her medical history and reproductive history. All these aspects must be taken into account in individual circumstances.

For women with mild to moderate depression without a history of recurrent or severe depression or women with depression related to specific adjustments or stressors, psychotherapy with a trained provider may be sufficient.

However, if the woman's history indicates a need for an antidepressant, because of symptoms severity, illness recurrences, or lack of access to psychotherapy, then a thorough risk-benefit discussion of antidepressants in general and the specific medications is warranted. Women considering use of SSRIs during pregnancy may weight any greater risk of premature delivery against the risk of persistent of recurrent depression and the availability and acceptability of alternative treatment (Chaudron, L, 2013).

Collaboration with the patient's obstetrician and even her pediatrician may be especially helpful in supporting the mother, and the psychiatrist in making an informed decision and following through on it.

Mothers can be anxious about initiating and continuing medications during pregnancy, but they may be just as anxious about discontinuing them or not starting them if they have experienced depression in the past and know that their symptoms interfere with their lives. Working with the pregnant woman and her support structure to understand what is known, what is unknown, the risks, and the benefits of the whole picture will lead to a truly informed decision that will allow the mother to feel that she has made the best choice for her individual situation (Galbally, M, et al. 2016).

Neonatal Complications of Antidepressant Medication in Pregnancy

Many women will not contemplate taking medication during pregnancy, because of fears that it could harm the developing fetus and a significant number stop taking antidepressants in the first trimester of pregnancy. As a consequence, depression will persist and could have an adverse effect on pregnancy outcome. However, the women on antidepressants may experience significant side effects from the medication, and effects of the medications on obstetric outcome, and a possible risk of gestational hypertension. The major adverse effects of antidepressant medications in pregnancy include fetal malformations, persistent pulmonary hypertension, and poor neonatal adaptation syndrome (Oberlander TF, et al. 2006).

Of eight meta-analyses, four have found no association between antidepressant exposure and malformation. Three have found an association between paroxetine and heart defects (Wurst, KE, et al. 2010). Two recent meta-analyses also found an association between fluoxetine and an increased malformation risk. Both tricyclic antidepressants (TCAs) and the Selective Noradrenaline Reuptake Inhibitors (SNRIs) have not been associated with malformation, however studies are limited. Confounding variables are important, given that women with mental illness, including depression, have higher rates of vitamin deficiencies, such as vitamin D, poorer nutrition, obesity and deficit in folate. The latter is significant as folate is essential to prevent malformations such as neural tube defects, but also potentially for cardiac malformation.

Whether depression or anxiety, are in themselves, teratogenic, and therefore associated with structural or neurodevelopmental teratogenicity, is still unconfirmed.

The basic premise of teratology is that exposure during early pregnancy to a specific agent results in a specific malformation. While there is concerning data about a potential small increase in malformation risk from exposure to antidepressants in pregnancy, particularly specific SSRIs such as paroxetine, there have not been conclusive results about this risk (Grigoriadis, S, et al. 2013).

Persistent Pulmonary hypertension of the Newborn (PPHN) has been reported in several studies investigating the potential association between SSRI, TCA and SNRIS exposure in pregnancy. They found a general incidence of PPHN of 1.2 per 1,000 and with exposure this increased to 3 per 1,000 (Grigoriadis, S, et al. 2014).

Teratogenic Risk of Psychotropic Medications

All psychotropic agents cross the placenta to some degree and are excreted in the mother's milk during breastfeeding. This puts both doctor and patient in a very unpleasant bind. Ideally, every mother should be totally drug free throughout every pregnancy. However, there are many instances in which the known risks of discontinuing psychiatric medications are greater than the unknown risks of continuing to take them.

Not treating mental illness during pregnancy has significant risks. Severely depressed pregnant women do not take care of themselves optimally, and studies have suggested a higher risk of low birth weight and preterm delivery in untreated depressed women. When the risk of suicide is added to the equation, the risk can escalate further.

As far as we can determine, the only drugs commonly used in psychiatry with proven relationships to specific birth defects are lithium, most anticonvulsants, paroxetine and benzodiazepines.

Documented informed consent from the patient and her family (including her husband or her parents, when appropriate) for the treatment plan is necessary, whether one decides to leave the patient drug free with the risks of that course or to continue with a needed medication despite the pregnancy.

Is it likely that stopping most psychotropic medication 2-3 weeks before the pregnancy is early enough to avoid fetus malformation. If medication can be avoided for the first 3 months of pregnancy, the risk of fetal abnormality is much reduced, but other risks can occur. Babies born to mothers who are physically dependent on sedatives suffer withdrawal symptoms and need to be treated postnatally. Autonomic withdrawal symptoms presumably can occur in the newborn if the mother has been taking tricyclic antidepressants (TCAs) or short acting antidepressants such as paroxetine and venlafaxine (Yonkers, KA, et al. 2009). However, the risk of the fetus/newborn may be small relative to the risks posed by not treating a vulnerable woman as she begins the postpartum period.

Overall, antidepressants are probably the best-studied class of agents during pregnancy relative to all other medicines. The most recent data and reviews on fluoxetine exposure during pregnancy suggest that fluoxetine is not associated with a higher rate of birth anomalies. More than 5,000 women in a national database who were taking fluoxetine have been prospectively studied, and there is no clear evidence of teratogenic effects for fluoxetine. However, there has been an association of SSRIs exposure in pregnancy with higher rates of spontaneous abortions, a self-limiting neonatal behavioral syndrome characterized by motor effects, irritability, and gastrointestinal upset, and possible even a small risk of postnatal pulmonary hypertension (Schatzberg, Alan F., and Charles DeBattista 2015).

All SSRIs except paroxetine are currently considered under the U.S Food and Drug Administration (FDA), as having the risk of teratogen effects cannot be ruled out because of insufficient evidence. The known risk with bupropion is less than of the SSRIs. Although animal studies on bupropion may suggest minimal risk of teratogenic effects, there are virtually no clinical data. Thus, use bupropion over an SSRI in pregnancy cannot be confirmed.

Likewise, some TCAs such as nortriptyline per FDA suggest that there is positive evidence of risk. For patients who have clearly responded to nortriptyline, it may be much safer for them to continue the drug than to switch to a SSRI.

Benzodiazepines were traditionally considered to be contraindicated in pregnancy. Many of them according to FDA, indicated that the teratogenic risks of these agents generally outweigh the potential benefits, and are therefore contraindicated. The concern was that first trimester exposure was associated with an increased risk of cleft palate and cleft lip.

Anxiety Disorders

Regarding panic disorder, pregnancy has for a long time been believed to be protective, which has, however, not been supported by a prospective study. The onset or worsening of OCD during pregnancy has also been frequently described. Symptoms of all anxiety disorders can be so severe that in some cases patients even consider an interruption of the pregnancy because they feel that cannot bear the symptoms until delivery and/or the fear of medication adverse effects on the unborn. Furthermore, anxiety during pregnancy has been associated with an increased incidence of perinatal complications and postpartum depression.

MANAGEMENT OF ANXIETY DISORDERS IN PREGNANCY

Women with antenatal anxiety disorders require timely and efficient management that aims to reduce all such symptoms that may adversely impact on baby's health.

NON-PHARMACOLOGICAL INTERVENTIONS

Alternative interventions to pharmacological treatments should be considered first line options. Mild to moderate symptoms of anxiety are highly treatable using Cognitive Behavioral Therapy (CBT), an evidence-based, short-term, and focused treatment, in which patients learn to identify their distorted thinking, increase awareness of triggers, and modify maladaptive behaviors. Stress reduction techniques such as meditation, modified deep breathing for pregnant women, and exercising may complement other forms of treatment. Similarly, treatment such as biofeedback and acupuncture show promise, but their effectiveness is not conclusive. Another treatment is music therapy, a safe and inexpensive method to reduce antenatal anxiety (Wiegartz and Gyoerkoe 2009; Avni-Barron 2001). Preliminary information seems to suggest that both massage, and aromatherapy may be successful in producing clinically significant reductions in anxiety.

BENZODIAZEPINES

When possible, benzodiazepines (BDZ's) should be avoided in both the first trimester and third trimester of pregnancy due to possible structural teratogenicity (anal atresia, and oral cleft), spontaneous abortion, and neonatal withdrawal syndromes (Bellantuono, C., et al. 2013).To minimize the risk of neonatal withdrawal, BDZs should be tapered gradually before delivery, tapering should begin 3-4 weeks before the due date and BDZ treatment should be discontinued at least 1 week before delivery (Vythilingum, B, 2008).

Table 1. Summary of antenatal anxiety and major depression

- The rates of mood disorders in women are approximately equivalent in pregnant and non- childbearing women.
- Prevalence rate between 3 and 9%.
- Pregnancy and puerperium are important life transitions.
- Maternal health is considered for the World Health Organization a global priority.
- Making a diagnosis of major depressive disorder in pregnancy is complicated by the fact that there are overlapping symptoms between major depression and pregnancy related symptoms.
- Mild to moderate anxiety disorder or MDD can be treated with psychotherapy.
- When possible, avoid first trimester exposure to antidepressants and standing benzodiazepine combinations.
- When the patient is willing to and the depression is severe, continue antidepressants. Do not stop antidepressant abruptly. In case of discontinuation, taper the dosage.
- Treat to remission. Use the lowest effective dosage.
- There has been an association of SSRIs exposure in pregnancy with higher rates of spontaneous abortions, a self-limiting "neonatal behavioral syndrome" characterized by motor effects, irritability, gastrointestinal upset, and possibly even a small risk of postnatal pulmonary hypertension.
- Alternative treatments: exercise, mindfulness, relaxation, acupuncture, herbal remedies, exercise, or relaxation and bright light therapy.

PREGABALIN

Since no information is available about the outcomes of pregnancies exposed to pregabalin, the drug should be avoided during pregnancy.

Hypnotic Benzodiazepine Receptor Agonist

Preliminary data, although apparently encouraging, are too limited to confirm or exclude a potential structural teratogenic liability. However, use should be discouraged, because of an increase in the risk of gestational teratogenicity (preterm birth, low birth weight, and babies that are small for their gestational age).

Antidepressants

Antidepressants have been shown to be an effective treatment for a range of anxiety disorders including General Anxiety Disorder.

References

Bellantuono, Cesario, Stefania Tofani, Guido Di Sciascio, and Giovanni Santone. "Benzodiazepine exposure in pregnancy and risk of major malformations: a critical overview." *General hospital psychiatry* 35, no. 1 (2013): 3-8.

Cohen, Lee S., Lori L. Altshuler, Bernard L. Harlow, Ruta Nonacs, D. Jeffrey Newport, Adele C. Viguera, Rita Suri et al. "Relapse of major depression during pregnancy in women who maintain or discontinue antidepressant treatment." *JAMA* 295, no. 5 (2006): 499-507.

Chaudron, Linda H. "Complex challenges in treating depression during pregnancy." *American Journal of Psychiatry* 170, no. 1 (2013): 12-20.

Einarson, Adrienne, Peter Selby, and Gideon Koren. "Discontinuing antidepressants and benzodiazepines upon becoming pregnant. Beware of the risks of abrupt discontinuation." *Canadian Family Physician* 47, no. 3 (2001): 489-490.

Flynn, Heather A., Frederic C. Blow, and Sheila M. Marcus. "Rates and predictors of depression treatment among pregnant women in hospital-affiliated obstetrics practices." *General hospital psychiatry* 28, no. 4 (2006): 289-295.

Galbally, Megan, Martien Snellen, and Andrew Lewis. *Psychopharmacology and Pregnancy*. Springer-Verlag Berlin An, 2016.

Gyoerkoe, Kevin, and Pamela Wiegartz. *The pregnancy and postpartum anxiety workbook: Practical skills to help you overcome anxiety, worry, panic attacks, obsessions, and compulsions*. New Harbinger Publications, 2009.

Grigoriadis, Sophie, Emily H. VonderPorten, Lana Mamisashvili, George Tomlinson, Cindy-Lee Dennis, Gideon Koren, Meir Steiner, Patricia Mousmanis, Amy Cheung, and Lori E. Ross. "Prenatal exposure to antidepressants and persistent pulmonary hypertension of the newborn: systematic review and meta-analysis." *BMJ* 348 (2014): f6932.

Grigoriadis, Sophie, Emily H. VonderPorten, Lana Mamisashvili, Allison Eady, George Tomlinson, Cindy-Lee Dennis, Gideon Koren et al. "The effect of prenatal antidepressant exposure on neonatal adaptation: a systematic review and meta-analysis." (2013): e309-20.

Halbreich, Uriel. "Prevalence of mood symptoms and depressions during pregnancy: implications for clinical practice and research." *CNS spectrums* 9, no. 3 (2004): 177-184.

Myles, Nicholas, Hannah Newall, Harvey Ward, and Matthew Large. "Systematic meta-analysis of individual selective serotonin reuptake inhibitor medications and congenital malformations." *Australian & New Zealand Journal of Psychiatry* 47, no. 11 (2013): 1002-1012.

Oberlander, Tim F., William Warburton, Shaila Misri, Jaafar Aghajanian, and Clyde Hertzman. "Neonatal outcomes after prenatal exposure to selective serotonin reuptake inhibitor antidepressants and maternal depression using population-based linked health data." *Archives of general psychiatry* 63, no. 8 (2006): 898-906.

Riecher-Rössler, Anita, and Meir Steiner, eds. *Perinatal stress, mood and anxiety disorders: from -bench to bedside*. Vol. 173. Karger Medical and Scientific Publishers, 2005.

Schatzberg, Alan F., and Charles DeBattista. *Manual of clinical psychopharmacology*. American Psychiatric Pub, 2015.

Ververs, Tessa, Hans Kaasenbrood, Gerard Visser, Fred Schobben, Lolkje de Jong-van den Berg, and Toine Egberts. "Prevalence and patterns of antidepressant drug use during pregnancy." *European journal of clinical pharmacology* 62, no. 10 (2006): 863-870.

Vythilingum, Bavanisha. "Anxiety disorders in pregnancy." *Current psychiatry reports* 10, no. 4 (2008): 331-335.

Weissman, Myrna M., and Mark Olfson. "Depression in women: implications for health care research." *Science* 269, no. 5225 (1995): 799-801.

Wurst, Keele E., Charles Poole, Sara A. Ephross, and Andrew F. Olshan. "First trimester paroxetine use and the prevalence of congenital, specifically cardiac, defects: a meta-analysis of epidemiological studies." *Birth Defects Research Part A: Clinical and Molecular Teratology* 88, no. 3 (2010): 159-170.

Yonkers, Kimberly A., Katherine L. Wisner, Donna E. Stewart, Tim F. Oberlander, Diana L. Dell, Nada Stotland, Susan Ramin, Linda Chaudron, and Charles Lockwood. "The management of depression during pregnancy: a report from the American Psychiatric Association and the American College of Obstetricians and Gynecologists." *General hospital psychiatry* 31, no. 5 (2009): 403-413.

Yonkers, Kimberly A., Megan V. Smith D Ph, Haliqun Lin, Heather B. Howell, Lin Shao, and Robert A. Rosenheck. "Depression screening of perinatal women: an evaluation of the healthy start depression initiative." *Psychiatric Services* 60, no. 3 (2009): 322-328.

Yonkers, Kimberly A., Nathan Gotman, Megan V. Smith, Ariadna Forray, Kathleen Belanger, Wendy L. Brunetto, Haiqun Lin, Ronald T. Burkman, Carolyn M. Zelop, and Charles J. Lockwood. "Does antidepressant use attenuate the risk of a major depressive episode in pregnancy?" *Epidemiology* (Cambridge, Mass.) 22, no. 6 (2011): 848.

In: Women's Pearls
Editors: S. Fink and P. Korenis
ISBN: 978-1-53616-103-8

Chapter 6

UNDERSTANDING AND ENSURING POSTPARTUM HEALTH

Mihir Upadhyaya, MD, PhD*
Bronx-Care Health System,
Icahn School of Medicine at Mount Sinai, New York, NY, US

INTRODUCTION

Nothing in medicine is more natural or joyous than the beginning of a human life, and the roles that people assume as new mothers, fathers, and caretakers. Consequently, no part of the human experience is more life-altering than accepting the responsibility of parenthood. For a new mother, it is a dynamic period full of changes and adjustments in lifestyle and responsibility, in addition to physical and mental health. The volume of change during the postpartum period renders it the most vulnerable times in a woman's life. Unfortunately, postpartum health is among the least-researched, most-neglected aspects of women's health care, particularly as it pertains to mental health. The amplified attention in recent years on the

* Corresponding Author's E-mail: mupadhya@bronxleb.org.

dire consequences of postpartum mental illness has increased the need for addressing this phase of motherhood.

Postpartum Period

Clinically, the postpartum period is often divided into three distinct but continuous phases, starting from the time of delivery and typically lasting up to six months (Romano et al., 2010).

The initial postpartum phase, or acute phase, involves the first 6-12 hours after delivery. This is a time of rapid and dynamic physiological change, and new mothers are monitored closely for complications such as postpartum hemorrhage, uterine inversion, amniotic fluid embolism, and eclampsia. The second postpartum phase, also called the subacute phase, starts immediately after the first phase, and can typically last 2-6 weeks after delivery. During this time, the new mother's body undergoes major changes in hemodynamics, genitourinary recovery, and metabolism. This is also a time of considerable changes in endocrinology, when hormones such as estrogen and progesterone, which were at high levels in the mother's body to maintain pregnancy, suddenly plummet back to the levels of a normal non-pregnant woman in a matter of days. The third postpartum phase, known as the delayed phase, starts after the second phase and can last up to six months after delivery. Changes during this phase include gradual restoration of muscle tone and connective tissue to the pre-pregnant state.

The arduous process of pregnancy and delivery combined with the multitude of physiological and hormonal changes that occur in a new mother's body after childbirth, and the subsequent responsibilities a new mother must assume in her new role can all contribute to a cluster of psychiatric conditions that, if not identified and treated, could pose dire consequences.

Psychiatric issues arising shortly after childbirth often fall into a multitude of distinct diagnoses: the "baby blues," postpartum depression, postpartum anxiety, postpartum post-traumatic stress disorder, and postpartum psychosis.

The "Baby Blues"

Somewhere between 50 - 80% of new mothers are believed to be affected by the "baby blues," the symptoms of which include anxiety and nervousness, sadness or feelings of loss, irritability, bouts of crying or tearfulness, mood swings, difficulty concentrating, trouble sleeping, vivid fantasies or dreams, excessive fatigue, desire for isolation, and a lack of motivation to perform activities of daily living, including adhering to proper hygiene and eating (M'Bailara et al., 2005). These symptoms typically start 1 to 3 days after delivery and last for 1 to 2 weeks. Symptoms are intermittent and can be aggravated by stressors such as breastfeeding, pain, discomfort from physical exertion, or social interaction.

Table 1. Symptoms of the "Baby Blues"

Signs and symptoms of baby blues — which last only a few days to a week or two after your baby is born — may include: • Mood swings • Anxiety • Sadness • Irritability • Feeling overwhelmed • Crying • Reduced concentration • Appetite problems • Trouble sleeping

The "baby blues" are more prevalent after high-risk deliveries, when maternal health is compromised during the latter stages of pregnancy and subsequent childbirth, in situations where the newborn infant is in sub-optimal health, or in scenarios where the new mother perceives a lack of social support or empathy. This phenomenon is thought to be a natural part of the physiological and emotional adjustment following childbirth, and it does not compromise the new mother's ability to take care of herself or the newborn. Symptoms typically resolve without formal treatment.

POSTPARTUM DEPRESSION

In some cases, the "baby blues" persist for longer than the expected course of time, and they may even increase in severity. When this happens, the condition is classified as postpartum depression, which happens to be the most common complication of childbearing, affecting approximately 13% of new mothers (O'Hara & Swain, 1996). Meanwhile, prevalence among teenage mothers is thought to be 26%. The condition usually begins within the first four weeks following delivery, and most cases require treatment by a health care professional. The depression may be a continuation of "baby blues," or can occur as a gradual onset, days to weeks after delivery, after a period of well-being. Recently published epidemiological literature suggests that mood disturbances following childbirth are not significantly different from depression that may occur at any other point in life. However, postpartum depression receives its own classification in the Diagnostic and Statistical Manual of Mental Disorders, 5th Edition (DSM-5), because the symptoms are focused on the adjustment process that begins at delivery, and the impact of this specific form of depression on the mother and infant.

Postpartum depression is characterized by tearfulness, hopelessness, mood swings, feelings of guilt, loss of appetite, suicidal ideation, difficulty sleeping, poor concentration and memory, fatigue, feelings of inadequacy, and inability to cope with the responsibility of caring for the baby. Some new mothers worry excessively about the baby's health or feeding habits and seem themselves as inadequate or unloving. To meet the diagnostic criteria for postpartum depression, symptoms must be continuously present for at least 2 weeks and interfere with the mother's ability to perform her normal activities of daily living, which, in the case of new mothers, also include taking care of the baby.

While the symptoms of postpartum depression are the same as depression occurring at other times, distinguishing between depressive symptoms and the typical sequelae of childbirth, such as post-delivery weight loss, changes in sleep patterns to accommodate the needs of the baby, and fatigue from the added responsibilities of childcare, and the calorie demands of milk production, may be a challenge that complicates clinical diagnosis. While severe postpartum depression may be obvious, lesser-acute presentations can be dismissed as a normal or natural part of the aftermath of childbirth. Failure to recognize postpartum mood disturbances can sometimes result in tragic consequences for the mother and baby, notably maternal suicide and infanticide.

Most postpartum depression is self-limiting and resolves within weeks to months after onset. However, for many women, the act of birthing a baby serves as a stressor that triggers the start of recurrent or chronic episodes of depression. Women who experience postpartum depression are at risk of suffering further episodes of illness, both following subsequent deliveries and at times unrelated to childbirth. For new mothers who suffer from postpartum depression, the risk of recurrence of major depression at another time in their life is 25%.

POSTPARTUM ANXIETY

This is a condition experienced by nearly 6% of expectant mothers during some phase of their pregnancy, and 10% of new mothers during the postpartum period (Wenzel et al., 2005). It may occur on its own, or in addition to postpartum depression or another psychiatric condition. Women at highest risk for postpartum anxiety are those with a personal or family history of anxiety, previous history of depression, or women found to have a thyroid imbalance.

New mothers with postpartum anxiety may have difficulty sleeping or not have an appetite. They might experience dizziness or nausea, or uncomfortable skin flushing. It may be uncomfortable to sit still for extended periods of time. They can constantly worry, not just about their own health or that of their baby, but about matters outside their scope of involvement or control. They could experience racing thoughts, where they're inundated with the same recurrent idea, or engulfed by different lines of thought they find intrusive, distracting, or overwhelming.

Table 2. Symptoms of postpartum depression

Postpartum depression may be mistaken for baby blues at first — but the signs and symptoms are more intense and last longer, and may eventually interfere with your ability to care for your baby and handle other daily tasks. Symptoms usually develop within the first few weeks after giving birth, but may begin earlier — during pregnancy — or later — up to a year after birth. Postpartum depression signs and symptoms may include: • Depressed mood or severe mood swings • Excessive crying • Difficulty bonding with your baby • Withdrawing from family and friends • Loss of appetite or eating much more than usual • Inability to sleep (insomnia) or sleeping too much • Overwhelming fatigue or loss of energy • Reduced interest and pleasure in activities you used to enjoy • Intense irritability and anger • Fear that you're not a good mother • Hopelessness • Feelings of worthlessness, shame, guilt or inadequacy • Diminished ability to think clearly, concentrate or make decisions • Restlessness • Severe anxiety and panic attacks • Thoughts of harming yourself or your baby • Recurrent thoughts of death or suicide Untreated, postpartum depression may last for months or longer.

Table 3. Symptoms of postpartum anxiety

This is a condition experienced by nearly 6% of expectant mothers during some phase of their pregnancy, and 10% of new mothers during the postpartum period (Wenzel et al., 2005). It may occur on its own or in addition to postpartum depression or another psychiatric condition. Symptoms may include: • Increase heart rate • Stomach pains • Tightness in the chest or throat • Rapid breathing • Loss of appetite • Irritability • Difficulty falling or staying asleep • Racing thoughts about the future • Imagining the worst-case scenario • Worrying and obsessing • Avoiding certain situations, activities, places, or people • Over-controlling or micro-managing • Constantly seeking reassurance from others • Checking things repeatedly • Being extra careful and vigilant of danger • Muscle tension (grinding teeth, neck and shoulder pain, back pain, muscle twitching

In some cases, new mothers may have a specific form of postpartum anxiety known as postpartum panic disorder, where they experience panic attacks. These are instances when the affected person experiences shortness of breath, chest pain, heart palpitations, dizziness, claustrophobia, numbness and tingling in the arms and legs, and a general feeling of impending doom. Panic attacks tend to come in waves, can be set off by a known stimulus, or may occur without a particular reason. While they can be frightening, panic attacks tend to pass within a matter of seconds, and they do not leave lasting effects or pose a danger to physical health.

Postpartum anxiety is temporary and highly treatable with professional help. It is rare for the condition to require hospitalization or prolonged use of medication, though such measures must remain an option. Most issues involving anxiety after delivery are handled with supportive care and use of as-needed medication.

POSTPARTUM POST-TRAUMATIC STRESS DISORDER

Though it is not a diagnosis formally recognized in the DSM-5, up to 6% of women experience postpartum post-traumatic stress disorder (PTSD) after childbirth (Beck, 2004). The condition is caused by either an actual or perceived trauma during delivery, or shortly thereafter. Symptoms of the condition may include re-experiencing the perceived trauma of childbirth through recollections, flashbacks or nightmares, emotional numbness, avoidance of places, people, or activities that remind the mother of the trauma, hypervigilance, difficulty sleeping, poor concentration, or being easily irritated or angered. Among the most common incidents that may precipitate symptoms of postpartum PTSD include an unexpected pre-term delivery, unplanned C-section, use of vacuum extraction or forceps to deliver the baby, a prolapsed umbilical cord, or complications requiring the newborn to be in the neonatal intensive care unit. Women who experience physical complications or injury related to pregnancy or childbirth, including severe hemorrhage, unexpected hysterectomy, severe preeclampsia/eclampsia, perineal trauma (third or fourth degree tearing), or cardiovascular issues are also at higher risk for postpartum PTSD, as are women who experienced previous trauma such as rape or sexual abuse.

Symptoms of postpartum PTSD include intrusive thoughts, flashbacks, or nightmares causing the new mother to re-experience the traumatic event. Affected women might avoid stimuli associated with the event, including suppression of unpleasant thoughts, feelings, and memories, and avoidance of people and places associated with the trauma. Inability to escape negative stimuli might lead to anxiety or panic attacks. The new mother may also experience a persistent feeling of increased arousal, including irritability, difficulty sleeping, hypervigilance, or being easily startled. She may feel a sense of unreality or detachment, which may compromise her ability to care for herself and her baby.

Table 4. Symptoms of postpartum post-traumatic stress disorder

Though it is not a diagnosis formally recognized in the DSM-5, up to 6% of women experience postpartum post-traumatic stress disorder after childbirth. Symptoms may include:

- Re-experiencing the perceived trauma of childbirth through recollections, flashbacks, and nightmares.
- Emotional numbness
- Avoidance of places, people, and activities that are reminders of the trauma
- Hypervigilance
- Difficult sleeping
- Poor concentration
- Being easily irritated or angered

Postpartum PTSD is temporary and highly treatable with professional help. Depending on the severity of symptoms, the appropriate treatment plan may include supportive care, a short-term course of medication, or brief hospitalization.

POSTPARTUM PSYCHOSIS

The rarest, and perhaps most serious, psychiatric condition affecting new mothers is postpartum psychosis, which is estimated to affect mothers in 1 or 2 out of every 1000 births (Spinelli, 2009). The condition is a psychiatric emergency that requires prompt attention by a health care professional. Like psychosis that occurs at any other point in a person's life, it implies the afflicted person is operating outside the scope of reality. The onset of postpartum psychosis can be sudden, typically occurring within the first two weeks after delivery, though it may occur at any time during the first six months.

The symptoms of postpartum psychosis include paranoid delusions, which are false or irrational beliefs not based in reality or fact. In most cases, these beliefs are centered around the baby, the spouse/partner, or the mother's own health. Common delusions include ideations that the baby was switched at birth, or the spouse/partner is being unfaithful. A new mother with postpartum psychosis may experience rapid mood swings, where they alternate from feeling energetic and powerful to depressed and anxious, typically several times and a day. They may begin to hallucinate, hearing sounds or voices that aren't really there, seeing people or objects that don't exist, or feeling sensations on their skin or inside their body that have no stimulus. They might also get confused about how to perform familiar activities. Other common symptoms include difficulty sleeping, hyper- or hypoactivity, agitation, exhibiting unusual or bizarre behavior, or illogical thinking. Nearly 10% of mothers with postpartum psychosis may even have dangerous thoughts about harming themselves or their baby, and in rare instances, the condition has led to suicide or infanticide.

Table 5. Symptoms of postpartum psychosis

With postpartum psychosis — a rare condition that typically develops within the first week after delivery — the signs and symptoms are severe. Signs and symptoms may include:

- Confusion and disorientation
- Obsessive thoughts about your baby
- Hallucinations and delusions
- Sleep disturbances
- Excessive energy and agitation
- Paranoia
- Attempts to harm yourself or your baby

Postpartum psychosis may lead to life-threatening thoughts or behaviors and requires immediate treatment.

While the symptoms of postpartum psychosis are complex and varied, the condition has been stigmatized in recent years, largely from the way it has been portrayed in the media, which often over-emphasizes, exaggerates, and dramatizes the most extreme features and examples of the condition, particularly the ways in which new mothers harm themselves and their babies. These stigmas cause many to feel reluctance in seeking help, believing that admitting to symptoms of postpartum psychosis may lead to embarrassment, loss of reputation, or cause them to be forcibly separated from their baby.

While a new mother can fully recover from an acute episode of postpartum psychosis, the condition is closely linked to bipolar disorder, and 75 - 80% of women will go on to require treatment for this more-common psychiatric condition. Conversely, 25 - 50% of new mothers already diagnosed with bipolar disorder prior to delivery are predicted to experience postpartum psychosis. Women who experience this condition have a greater than 50% chance of experiencing it again after subsequent deliveries.

TIPS FOR MAINTAINING GOOD POSTPARTUM MENTAL HEALTH

While it's important to identify disorders in postpartum mental health to ensure they are controlled and treated, the ideal approach is to not only try and prevent them from arising but also promote strategies to ensure that new mothers navigate the postpartum phase with joy and good health (Pantley, 2004).

Here is advice to help in this goal:

Slip into Motherhood, Gradually

Motherhood is a marathon, not a sprint. While the pregnancy may have lasted nine months, and your baby's birth took only a "moment", growing into the role of mother is a gradual progression that can't possibly happen that fast. This is the most transformative experience of your life, physically, mentally, and emotionally. Give yourself permission to slip into the role in whatever timeframe is most comfortable for you. Not only is it okay to focus on this new aspect of your life and make it your top priority, it's necessary. Never feel guilty or conflicted about your new focus, or the time it takes for you to incorporate your obligations as a mother into your other roles and responsibilities.

Talk to Experienced Parents

Communicate with your own parents, siblings, relatives, and friends who've also raised young children and can understand what you are feeling. You likely already know other women who've confronted postpartum issues, and hearing their experience might provide assurance that, for most women, this phase is temporary and will pass. Make a confidante of someone who knew you prior to pregnancy, whom you trust, who might encourage you to seek professional help if they believe you may need it.

Don't Isolate Yourself

Once you are physically able, and receive clearance from your health care provider, engage with people, places, and situations outside your home. Reorienting yourself with the world at large can be therapeutic, improve your mood and attitude, and give you valuable context into your new role as a mother. Reacquaint yourself with the mall, park, library, coffee shop, or whatever else you enjoy. You might enjoy them even more when you're filled with pride as strangers smile at you and your baby. Your baby might also enjoy the stimulation of being somewhere new.

Join a Support Group

Today, a multitude of support groups are available for new mothers, both in-person and online. They can be invaluable in helping you process your feelings about every aspect of motherhood. With a plethora of choices, be sure to find support groups that align with your values and beliefs about parenting. Remember that women may have different ideas about bonding, breastfeeding, nutrition, exercise, parental roles, visitors, caregivers, socializing, health care, and sexual activity following childbirth. What's acceptable to other new mothers may not be comfortable for you. Seek out new mothers with like-minded parenting beliefs, and share your own beliefs and experiences while drawing upon those of others.

Accept Help from Others

When family and friends say, "Let me know if I can do anything," they usually mean it. Most people are happy to help a new mother, and it's gratifying for others to feel they played some role in your transition into motherhood and in your baby's upbringing. Allow people to have this feeling. Permit others to run errands for you, watch your baby while you nap, take care of your older children if you have them, or help with cooking, cleaning, and other chores.

Tell Your Spouse/Partner How They Can Help

You aren't this baby's only parent, and it's important to your postpartum health that your baby is cared for through co-parenting with your spouse or partner. While their intentions might be good, they may not be sure of how to be helpful. It is important to guide your spouse or partner on what you need from them, both in the logistics of caring for you and the baby and in being receptive to hearing your thoughts and feelings throughout the postpartum phase. Remember to recognize this new baby is also a life-altering change for them and be mindful of their thoughts and needs during this period of adjustment. Your spouse or partner should be your biggest support and asset, as you are for them.

Make Time for Sleep

Sleep is not an optional luxury, it's an absolute necessity. Lack of sleep will enhance the feelings of depression, stress, and anxiety. The average adult requires seven to nine hours of sleep per night, and these needs are no different for new mothers. Make certain that sleep is a priority. Nap when the baby sleeps, go to bed early, and sleep in later in the morning whenever possible. If you are co-sleeping with a spouse or partner, plan to sleep in shifts, to ensure that both of you are getting sufficient sleep as you take care of your newborn. If you are concerned about your baby's sleep patterns, ask others for advice, or consult your health care provider.

Looks Don't Matter Right Now

Appearance is not a priority. Your only obligation as a new mother is to yourself, your baby, and the process of adjusting to motherhood. Don't waste your time and energy worrying about what you or your house look like. Most people can empathize with the massive transformation you've undergone, from becoming pregnant, to delivering a baby, to breastfeeding. They will certainly understand if your hair, makeup, or clothes aren't perfect. They will also understand if there's a little extra clutter or dust where you live.

Go Back to Work, When You're Ready

There are times when your home life is an escape from the stresses of work. Remember that it can also work in reverse. When you are physically and mentally ready, resume your job. Many new mothers consider it therapeutic to go back to work, and find they're better mothers when they resume their professional life. Having time outside your home, away from your baby, helps remind you of your own individuality, and focusing on work can improve self-esteem, elevate your mood, and broaden your perspective; all of which make you a better mother.

Exercise Regularly

Exercise is essential to postpartum recovery. In addition to helping shed pregnancy weight and toning abdominal muscles to regain your pre-baby body, an appropriate exercise regimen can boost energy, promote better sleep, relieve stress, and help prevent or minimize postpartum depression. Once cleared by your health care provider, you should aim to exercise at least 150 minutes per week, starting with light exercise including short walks and swimming. Literature published in recent years is in overwhelming favor of incorporating yoga, meditation, and breathing techniques into postpartum exercise regimens.

Eat Well, Eat Healthy

Proper nutrition is just as vital for postpartum health as it was for pregnancy. If you are breastfeeding, it's important to remember that lactation places high demands on the body, and decreased micronutrient stores can heighten postpartum depression risk. Most research indicates that lactating women require 500 calories in addition to what they consumed to maintain their weight prior to pregnancy. It's recommended that new mothers eat nutrient-rich foods that are high in collagen, continue to take prenatal vitamins to ensure against nutritional deficit, and drink sufficient water to prevent dehydration and fatigue.

Take Care of Yourself

The postpartum stage of motherhood is a challenging phase for which there is only one true resolution: time. During this phase of adjustment, take time out to engage in activities you enjoy. Remember that reading a book, painting your nails, talking on the phone, and going out to lunch with friends doesn't take away from being a great mother. It enhances motherhood. Communicate your feelings with your partner, family, and friends, particularly if the postpartum experience becomes stressful or overwhelming. If required, seek help from a health care provider.

Love Yourself

Having a baby and becoming a mother is among the greatest miracles and accomplishments in all humanity. Regardless of what else you achieve in life, it is unlikely you'll rank anything higher in importance or significance. Take pride in what you've accomplished, and remember to reflect on and enjoy the strong, capable, multi-faceted person you are becoming.

References

Beck, CT. Post-Traumatic Stress Disorder Due to Childbirth: The Aftermath. *Nursing Research*, 2004, 53(4), 216-224.

M'Bailara, K; Swendsen, J; Glatigny-Dallay, E; Dallay, D; Roux, D; Sutter, AL; Demontes-Mainard, J; Henry, C. Baby blues: characterization and influence of psycho-social factors. *L'Encephale*, 2005, 31(3), 331-336.

O'Hara, MW; Swain, AM. Rates and risk of postpartum depression—a meta -analysis. *International Review of Psychiatry*, 1996, 8(1), 37-54.

Pantley, E. *"Baby Blues." Gentle Baby Care: No-Cry, No-Fuss, No-Worry--Essential Tips for Raising Your Baby*, Contemporary Books, 2004, pp. 9–16.

Romano, M; Cacciatore, A; Giordano, R; La Rosa, B. Postpartum period: three distinct but continuous phases. *Journal of Prenatal Medicine*, 2010, 4(2), 22-25.

Spinelli, MG. Postpartum Psychosis: Detection of Risk and Management. *The American Journal of Psychiatry*, 2009, 166(4), 405-408.

Wenzel, A; Haugen, EN; Jackson, LC; Brendel, JR. Anxiety symptoms and disorders at eight weeks postpartum. *Journal of Anxiety Disorders*, 2005, 19(3), 295-311.

In: Women's Pearls
Editors: S. Fink and P. Korenis
ISBN: 978-1-53616-103-8

Chapter 7

Psychopharmacology during Pregnancy and Lactation

Jean Daniel Mello, MD
Bronx-Care Hospital,
Icahn School of Medicine at Mount Sinai, New York, NY, US

Factors Affecting Drug Choice in Pregnancy

The concept of pregnancy as a time of emotional well-being and stability has recently been revisited—with current overwhelming evidence that pregnancy is not a protective factor for women with mental illness. Women, who abruptly discontinue their medications, during pregnancy or at any time, are a particularly vulnerable population. A study investigating the relapse rate of major depression during pregnancy in women who maintain or discontinue antidepressant treatment found that approximately one-quarter of women who maintained antidepressant treatment throughout pregnancy relapsed compared with over two-thirds of those who discontinued medication (Cohen, Altshuler, Harlow, Nonacs et al., 2006, pp. 499-507). Bipolar disorder is another example where significantly high rates of relapse are seen with discontinuation of medication as compared to pharmacological maintenance.

Clearly, however, there can be no guarantee of a successful outcome in any pregnancy. Risks are inherent to life, and pregnancy is no exception. Spontaneous abortion in early pregnancy occurs in approximately 10-20% of pregnant women and baseline risk of spontaneous congenital malformation is approximately 2-4%. When a negative outcome in pregnancy arises, it should not be automatically assumed that prescription medication was the causative agent.

Multiple factors have an influence on pregnancy outcome including smoking, alcohol consumption and a poor diet. Pre-pregnancy obesity has been recently associated with increased risk of neural tube defects. In fact, untreated psychiatric illness itself has been shown to adversely affect pregnancy and result in birth-related outcomes. Depression and anxiety are two psychiatric illnesses with the highest prevalence during pregnancy. Complications related to maternal mental illness include low birth weight, fetal growth retardation, preterm delivery, increased risk of pre-eclampsia[1] and infant admission to a neonatal intensive care unit for conditions varying from respiratory distress, to hypoglycemia and prematurity.

All medications diffuse readily across the placenta, and as of yet, no psychotropic medication has been approved by the Food and Drug Administration (FDA) for use during pregnancy. Psychotropic medications are associated with potential risk including malformations (particularly with first-trimester exposure), neonatal toxicity (third-trimester exposure risk) as well as increased risk of subsequent longer-term neurobehavioral effects and physical health issues in adult age.

Scientific evidence on the safety of individual psychotropic medication during pregnancy is difficult to obtain due to ethical issues that make it difficult or impossible to conduct gold standard double blind trials in pregnant and lactating women. This ethical dilemma means that in practical terms, there is not sufficiently adequate and indisputable evidence on the safety or risks associated with specific medications. Research has mostly yielded results from case control studies from women who have been informed and have consented to taking medication during

---

[1] High blood pressure in patients who previously did not have the condition.

pregnancy/lactation. These results, however, may signify an underlying inherent bias in the sense that perhaps groups of women who agree to take medications during pregnancy/lactation are those with greatest risk factors and/or severity of psychiatric illness.

Women with histories of psychiatric illness frequently consult with psychiatrists during pregnancy. However, the majority of pregnancies in the U.S are unplanned, thereby occurring unexpectedly in women already receiving medications. Decisions regarding initiation or maintenance of psychotropic medication must be carefully assessed. Psychiatrists and pregnant women must make a balanced, individualized decision regarding treatment. The question becomes not one of risk versus benefit, but of risk versus risk, that is, the risk of exposure to medication for the mother/fetus versus the risk of exposure of mother/fetus to untreated illness.

ANTIDEPRESSANTS AND PREGNANCY: DEPRESSION DURING PREGNANCY AND POSTPARTUM

Depression during pregnancy is common. An estimated 10% of pregnant women will develop a depressive illness, with approximately one-third of cases of postpartum depression actually beginning before birth. Following delivery, women are at a significantly increased risk of developing new psychiatric episodes, particularly in the first three months after the birth of an infant. Around 80% of these episodes are mood disorders, with depression counting as the primary diagnosis. Those with a previous history of depressive illness at any point in time are at highest risk of additional episodes during pregnancy and in the postpartum period.

Antidepressants are the mainstay for treatment of moderate-to-severe depression in women. Guidelines specific to the perinatal period advocate that these medications be considered where there is a clear lack of response to psychosocial interventions or significant and debilitating symptoms of depression. It is essential that in all varying severity of depressive illness, lifestyle factors such as diet, exercise and sleep hygiene also be addressed with recommendations and clear goals. For mild-to-moderate depression, women should be initially offered psychosocial treatments including therapy of different modalities such as cognitive behavior therapy or interpersonal therapy. When pharmacotherapy is indicated, monotherapy (use of only one medication) should be preferred, using the lowest effective dose possible. However, it is of crucial importance that this dosage is sufficient enough so as to avoid suboptimal, partial treatment. Insufficient pharmacotherapy results in continued exposure to mother and child from risks of both treatment and illness.

The majority of antidepressants prescribed to women during pregnancy fall into the category of SSRIs—Selective Serotonin Re-Uptake Inhibitors, which appear not to be major teratogens (agents that cause malformation of the embryo or fetus). In the United States alone, approximately 10% of pregnant women are prescribed antidepressants, with the medication class of SSRIs as the overwhelming majority. Though an individualized case-by-case decision should always prevail, there are clear risks in not treating depression, both to the mother as well as to the fetus. These include harm to mother via lack of obstetric care, poor self-care or self-harm, as well as harm to the fetus or neonate as a result of neglect. Maternal depression has also been associated with inherent increased risks including premature delivery, low birth weight and gestational diabetes. Also of concern is that depression is associated with lower rates of breastfeeding.

SSRIs

Fluoxetine has the most data supporting its safety in pregnancy, while Sertraline appears to be associated with least placental exposure. With the exception of Paroxetine, several meta-analyses combining studies with exposures to SSRIs have not demonstrated increase in the risk of congenital malformations of children exposed. Paroxetine, however, has been associated with cardiac malformations such as atrial and ventricular septal defects (although it is important to note that other studies have not shown increased teratogenicity of Paroxetine).

Some concerns have been raised regarding late pregnancy, specifically third-trimester exposure to SSRIs. Most seriously, there is a possible association of SSRIs with persistent pulmonary hypertension of the newborn (PPHN) although the absolute risk is relatively small and may be less than previously reported. Again, it is important to note that not all studies support the finding of increased risk.

Transient Neonatal Distress Syndrome is associated with exposure to or withdrawal from antidepressants. Approximately 25% of infants exposed to SSRIs late in pregnancy may experience symptoms which include: restlessness, increased crying, tremors, and increased muscle tone. Although these symptoms may be worrying, fortunately, they are relatively benign and disappear after a few days typically without necessary medical intervention. Risk may be higher with antidepressants with short half-life such as Paroxetine and Venlafaxine.

Generally accepted recommendations with regard to depression include maintaining patients already receiving antidepressants and at high risk of relapse on the same medication during pregnancy and following delivery. Women who develop moderate or severe depression during pregnancy should be treated, as depression may pose a significant health risk to both the mother and child. In fact, there is evidence that depression increases risk of spontaneous abortion, low birth weight and pre-term delivery. Previously effective antidepressant should be considered, and, for untreated patients, Sertraline may be a good option.

OTHER ANTIDEPRESSANTS

SSRIs are the class of antidepressants most used in pregnancy. There are, however, other antidepressants that may be considered, including Tricyclic Antidepressants (TCAs). These have been widely used in pregnancy without apparent harm to the fetus. Among the TCAs, Desipramine and Nortriptyline are often preferred as they are less anticholinergic and less hypotension than others in the class.

Monoamine oxidase inhibitors (MAOIs) should be avoided in pregnancy due to possible risk of congenital malformations as well as risk of hypertensive crisis. Newer antidepressants such as Venlafaxine, Bupropion, Mirtazapine and Trazodone have less data supporting safety.

Bipolar Disorder and Mood Stabilizers

Pregnancy has been definitively shown not to be a protective factor for women with bipolar disorder. When mood stabilizing medications are discontinued, relapse rates have been shown to be high, with the majority of recurrences involving depressive episodes or dysphoric mixed states. The risk of relapse after delivery is particularly increased.

Bipolar disorder is also a significant risk factor for postpartum psychosis; therefore, mood stabilizing medication, the pharmacological gold standard for control of the disorder, is essential. However, these medications are not without risk, the most serious of which are the risks of teratogenicity. This issue raises a unique cause for concern since over 50% of pregnancies in the U.S are unplanned, particularly among women with bipolar disorder.

Anticonvulsants - Valproate, Carbamazepine, Lamotrigine

Of all medications used in psychiatry, Valproate is the one associated with greatest potential of birth defects, particularly neural tube defects including spina bifida. Prenatal exposure of Valproate has also been commonly associated with craniofacial malformations, cardiovascular abnormalities as well as limb and genital defects.

Valproate, Carbamazepine and Lamotrigine are medications classified as anticonvulsants and should be avoided during pregnancy unless absolutely necessary, particularly Valproate and Carbamazepine. They are considered teratogens. Exposure to Valproate is associated with neural tube defects ranging from 1-6% and is particularly teratogenic in early pregnancy, when many women are unaware of their pregnancy. In fact, the serious teratogenic profile of these medications has led many psychiatrists to absolutely contraindicate prescribing Valproate and Carbamazepine to women of child-bearing age.

Neonatal complications are most prevalent with Valproate with reports of fetal cardiac decelerations, hepatotoxicity (chemical-driven liver damage), and hypoglycemia as well as withdrawal symptoms in the newborn including feeling difficulties, irritability and abnormal muscle tone. Children exposed to Valproate have also been associated with poorer neurocognitive development. It should however be noted that Carbamazepine and Lamotrigine have not been associated with developmental delays and IQ reductions seen with Valproate.

Recently, there is growing evidence that Lamotrigine may be safer than Valproate and Carbamazepine although there may be a small increase in risk the of cleft lip or palate as compared to non-exposed children, an estimated increased absolute risk of around 0.9%.

Lithium

Lithium has been shown to distribute freely across the placenta, from mother to fetus, and should, if possible, be avoided in pregnancy. Its use is associated with fetal cardiac abnormality known as Ebstein's anomaly, though this risk has likely been overestimated, and more recent data suggest that risk of fetal malformation subsequent to lithium exposure to be between 0.05% and 0.1%, or between 1 in 2000 and 1 in 1000 (representing approximately 20-40 times the general population risk). Current available data regarding infant neurodevelopmental outcomes following in utero exposure to lithium indicate no identifiable difference between exposed and non-exposed infants.

There have, however, been cases where lithium has been the only medication a patient has responded to, in which case the benefits of continuing lithium outweigh the potential adverse consequences of decompensation and the risk that may ensue on the woman and child. In such cases, high-resolution ultrasound and echocardiography should be performed during pregnancy. If discontinuation of lithium is planned, slow tapering, ideally before pregnancy is recommended. The period of maximum risk to fetus has been estimated to be approximately 2-6 weeks after conception, a time before many women are aware of their pregnancy. It is important to note, however, that abrupt discontinuation is associated with further increased risks of relapse.

Anti-Anxiety Medications

Much discussion has occurred as to whether prenatal exposure to benzodiazepines increases the risk of organ malformation. A slightly increased risk of cleft lip or palate, calculated to be less than 1%, has been estimated. Third trimester use of benzodiazepines has however been associated with increased risk of neonatal withdrawal symptoms. Depending on the half-life of the benzodiazepine used, the symptoms can appear within a few days up to three weeks following birth. Benzodiazepine neonatal withdrawal symptoms include symptoms such as tremors, suckling difficulties, muscle tone disturbances, vomiting and diarrhea. Fortunately, most infants will recover without any long-lasting sequelae.

With regard to the non-benzodiazepine anxiolytic medications Buspirone and Pregabalin, as well as the hypnotic Z drugs such as Zolpidem and Zaleplon, the available data is at this time is scarce, and therefore these drugs are not recommended for use in pregnant women.

Anti-Psychotic Medication

The fact that psychiatric illness during pregnancy is in itself an independent risk factor for congenital malformations and perinatal mortality in individuals is well established. This background risk is certainly a confounding factor when assessing effects of antipsychotic medication. Women who present with a history of psychiatric disorders such as schizophrenia and who are maintained on antipsychotic medication should be encouraged to discuss plans to become pregnant as early as possible. Pregnancies of women with schizophrenia are considered high risk and reproductive health planning should be addressed in all women of reproductive age with serious mental illness.

In general terms, women who are stable on current antipsychotic medication and who are at high risk for relapse without medication should be advised to continue their current medication. Switching medication may be appropriate for some patients but are not generally recommended due to risk of relapse. Antipsychotics may also induce hyperprolactinemia,[2] which may in fact prevent pregnancy. Women who present with the condition may need to be switched to an alternative medication. An extensive cost-benefit discussion considering the antipsychotic medication that has worked best for the patient should occur. In addition, other risk factors for adverse outcomes such as substance use and smoking should routinely be addressed.

Antipsychotic medications are used to treat many differing psychiatric disorders ranging from psychotic disorders such as schizophrenia, bipolar disorder, as well as treatment resistant depression. They are generally regarded as being relatively safe in pregnancy. Indeed, many women with schizophrenia and related psychoses are at greatly increased risk of relapse if medication is stopped. Consequences of an acute psychotic episode can have potentially disastrous outcome for both mother and fetus; therefore, women likely to relapse should be continued on antipsychotic medication during pregnancy as well as in the postpartum period.

Antipsychotic medications are divided into two different classes or generations. First generation antipsychotics are dopamine blockers, which act on dopamine receptors in many different pathways in the brain, as well as on other receptors such as muscarinic, adrenergic, and histamine

---

[2] A condition of elevated serum prolactin. Prolactin is an amino acid protein produced in the cells of the pituitary gland. Its primary function is to enhance breast development during pregnancy and to induce lactation.

receptors. Second-generation antipsychotics (also called atypical antipsychotics) also block dopamine receptors, but what distinguishes them from first-generation agents is their ability to block serotonin receptors. These drugs are also known as serotonin-dopamine blockers. Second-generation antipsychotics in fact have higher affinity for serotonin receptors than dopamine receptors.

Most safety data are available for atypical antipsychotic or second-generation medication including Quetiapine, Risperidone, and Olanzapine, with more limited data for Aripiprazole, Clozapine and Ziprasidone. It should be noted that Quetiapine has a low rate of placental passage.

The discontinuation of antipsychotics may produce symptoms in newborns that include agitation, increased crying, and increased suckling. Although these symptoms are generally benign and without long-term sequelae, women should preferentially give birth in facilities with access to neonatal intensive care units as a safety precaution.

PREGNANCY AND BREASTFEEDING

It is widely recommended, if possible, that women breastfeed their infants for at least the first six months of life in view of well-established long term benefits on the child's physical and cognitive development.

In general, most antipsychotic medications should be continued in breastfeeding women to reduce risk of relapse of psychiatric disorders. Switching medication after birth is not recommended due to high risk of relapse. Avoiding decompensation of maternal mental illness is essential, and in the few notable exceptions where breastfeeding is contraindicated, the mother should be advised to bottle-feed her infant with formula.

Some general rules applicable to breastfeeding women include avoiding polypharmacy (use of multiple medications concomitantly), using the lowest effective dose and continuing the same treatment prescribed while pregnant. Special attention should be given to premature infants as well as infants with hepatic, renal, cardiac or neurological impairment who may be at a higher risk from exposure to medication. Infants naturally have decreased abilities for drug clearance and therefore should be carefully monitored for any unusual patterns in feeding, growth or development.

Antipsychotic Medications

Asenapine, Brexipiprazole, Cariprazine, Chlorpromazine, Clozapine, Haloperidol, Lloperidone, Lurasidone, Olanzapine, Paliperidone, Quetiapine, Risperidone, Ziprasidone

Clozapine use in breastfeeding mothers is deemed a risk significant for seizures and agranulocytosis[3] in infants; breastfeeding should not occur. Mothers should continue on Clozapine and infants should be bottle-fed with formula.

When initiation of an antipsychotic medication for postpartum psychosis is warranted, the medications Quetiapine and Olanzapine should be considered. Infant plasma concentration of these two medications in breastfeeding women has been shown to be undetectable or low.

Mood Stabilizers

Carbamazepine, Lamotrigine, Lithium, Topiramate, Valproate

Clinical practice dictates that mothers are prescribed mood stabilizers during pregnancy when benefits of continued treatment outweigh risk of discontinuation. In the postpartum period, it is advisable that the mood stabilizer used during pregnancy remain the same. This is not an optimal moment to consider switching for the purpose of breastfeeding.

Most mood stabilizers may be continued while breastfeeding occurs. The exception to this, however, is with Lithium. Mothers who are prescribed Lithium should not breastfeed due to possible Lithium

[3] A deficiency of granulocytes in the blood, causing increased vulnerability to infection.

intoxication in the infant. Mothers should continue Lithium and infants should be bottle-fed with formula.

When initiation of an antipsychotic mood stabilizing agent in the postpartum period is warranted, Quetiapine and Olanzapine should be considered. Infant plasma concentration of these two medications in breastfeeding women has been shown to be undetectable or low.

Antidepressant Medication

Agomelatine, Citalopram, Duloxetine, Escitalopram, Fluoxetine, Fluvoxamine, monoamine oxidase inhibitors (MAOIs), Mianserin, Mirtazapine, Moclobemide, Paroxetine, Reboxetine, Sertraline, Trazodone, Tricyclic antidepressants (TCAs), Venlafaxine, Vortioxetine.

Similarly to antipsychotic medication and mood stabilizers (with the exception of Lithium), it is not recommended to switch medication in the postpartum period for the purpose of breastfeeding. It is advisable to continue the medication used during pregnancy.

When initiation of an antidepressant for postpartum depression is warranted, Sertraline and Mirtazapine should be considered. Infant plasma concentration of these two medications in breastfeeding women has been shown to be undetectable or low.

Hypnotic Medication

Benzodiazepines, Zopiclone, Zolpidem, Zaleplon

Although generally best avoided, benzodiazepines with short half-life such as Lorazepam may be considered on an individual case-by-case basis.

Stimulant Medication

Atomoxetine, Dexamfetamine, Lisdexamfetamine, Methylphenidate

Similarly to antipsychotic medication and antidepressants, it is not recommended to switch medication in the postpartum period for the purpose of breastfeeding. It is advisable to continue the medication used during pregnancy.

SUMMARY

As we have read this chapter, pregnancy can be a highly challenging and stressful time for women in general, and particularly for women with underlying psychiatric disorders. Previously held notions of pregnancy being a period of psychiatric stability have recently been debunked with wide-spread acceptance that continued, ongoing assessment of women's mental health be maintained during pregnancy and in the postpartum period. Psychiatrists and their patients must carefully work together on an individual basis, discussing treatment options and pharmacological considerations. Strategies including maintaining, switching or discontinuing medication must be weighed against all other options in order to tailor treatment. During pregnancy and during the breastfeeding period, the question of risk of exposure to medication versus risk of exposure of mother and fetus/infant to untreated illness is of the utmost importance and must always be in the forefront of discussion between women and their treating psychiatrists.

Table 1. Recommendations - Psychotropic drugs during pregnancy

Treatment should always be tailored to the individual after careful consideration of current prescription, previous treatment response, and known risks of medication during pregnancy. Monotherapy, when possible, is preferred, in order to minimize the fetal exposure to medication.	
Medication	**Recommendations**
Antidepressants	• Women at high risk of relapse should ideally be maintained on the same antidepressant during and after pregnancy.
	• When initiating an antidepressant in a woman planning pregnancy, previous response to medication should be taken into account. Sertraline is an adequate option.
Antipsychotics	• There is no current and clear evidence that any antipsychotic is a major teratogen. • When initiating an antipsychotic during pregnancy or in a woman planning to become pregnant, previous response to medication should be taken into account. Switching is not routinely recommended. Quetiapine has a low rate of placental passage and is an adequate option. • Women should be screened for adverse metabolic effects. Oral glucose tolerance test should be offered. • Women taking antipsychotic medication should give birth in a facility with a neonatal intensive care unit.
Mood stabilizers	• Valproate should be discontinued in case of pregnancy. • Other anticonvulsants should ideally also be avoided (weigh risk and consequences of relapse against known risk of teratogenesis). • Lamotrigine is an option for bipolar depression only. • Consider mood stabilizing antipsychotic medication.
Sedatives	• Benzodiazepines, zolpidem and zopliclone are unlikely to be teratogenic, however, are best avoided in late pregnancy.

Table 2. Recommendations - Psychotropic drugs during breastfeeding

Drug Group	Recommended drugs
Antidepressants	• It is usually recommended to continue the medication that was used during pregnancy. It is not advisable to switch medication in the postpartum period for the purpose of breastfeeding. • When initiation of an antidepressant in the postpartum period is warranted, the medications Sertraline and Mirtazapine should be considered.
Antipsychotics	• It is usually recommended to continue the medication that was used during pregnancy. It is not advisable to switch medication in the postpartum period for the purpose of breastfeeding. • Clozapine use in breastfeeding women, however, should not occur. Mothers should continue on Clozapine and infant should be bottle-fed with formula. • When initiation of an antipsychotic in the postpartum period is warranted, the medications Olanzapine and Quetiapine should be considered.
Mood Stabilizers	• It is usually recommended to continue the medication that was used during pregnancy. It is not advisable to switch medication in the postpartum period for the purpose of breastfeeding. • Lithium use in breastfeeding women, however, should not occur. Mothers should continue on Lithium and infants should be bottle-fed with formula. • When initiation of a mood stabilizer in the postpartum period is warranted, the medications Olanzapine and Quetiapine should be considered.
Sedatives	• Generally best avoided. • Benzodiazepines with short half-life such as Lorazepam may be considered.

References

Cohen LS, Altshuler LL, Harlow BL, Nonacs R, et al. Relapse of major depression during pregnancy in women who maintain or discontinue antidepressant treatment. *JAMA*. 2006; 295(5):499-507.

Galbally M, Snellen M, Lewis A (Eds.). (2014). Psychopharmacology and pregnancy. *Treatment effficacy, risks and guidelines* (1st edition). Springer, Berlin-Heidelberg.

Sadock, B. J., Sadock, V. A., & Ruiz, P. (2017). *Kaplan & Sadock's comprehensive textbook of psychiatry* (10th edition). Philadelphia: Wolters Kluwer.

Stahl, S. M., & Grady, M. M. (2017). Stahl's Essential psychopharmacology: *The Prescriber's Guide* (6th edition). Cambridge, UK; Cambridge University Press.

Taylor, D.M., Barnes, T. R. E., Young, A. H. (2018). *The Maudsley Prescribing Guidelines in Psychiatry* (13th edition). Hoboken, NJ: Wiley-Blackwell.

In: Women's Pearls
Editors: S. Fink and P. Korenis
ISBN: 978-1-53616-103-8

Chapter 8

MENOPAUSE AND WOMEN'S MENTAL HEALTH

Monika Gashi*[*]*, MD
Bronx-Care Hospital,
Icahn School of Medicine at Mount Sinai, New York, NY, US

INTRODUCTION

Menopause is a pivotal phase in a woman's life. This phenomenon marks the cessation of the menstrual cycle, concluding the reproductive saga for women. The period preceding menopause is known as perimenopause which is characterized by the irregularity of menstrual cycles, which starts in mid to late 40's. By definition, a woman is in menopause after cessation of her menstrual periods for 12 consecutive months. The average age of menopause is about 51 years of age, but can range from 45-55 years of age. There are different etiologies of menstrual

[*] Corresponding Author's E-mail: MGashi@bronxleb.org.

cessation including: pregnancy, medical condition(s), medication induced, surgically induced and age-related menopause.

HISTORY

The term menopause comes from medical Latin word menopausis and Greek word men (menos) "month" and PIE root: me "to measure," and pausis "to cease, pause, stop." Dating back to antiquity, the Greek philosopher Aristotle noted in the 4th century that cessation of menses led to changes in emotion, unable to get pregnant, and weakness of health. Hippocrates associated menopause with breast cancer, but it was not until the 19th century when scientists started paying attention. During 1821, Charles Pierre Louis De Gardanne, a French physician, was the first person to coin the term menopause while studying women at great length and noting their symptoms as they aged. His work titled De la ménépausie, ou de l'âge critique des femmes which means "Menopause: the critical age of women." Was one of the first to emphasize changes throughout the lifecycle of a woman. During 1845 the French word menepausie was adopted to English language that now we know as Menopause. Initially, menopause carries with it a negative connotation. During this time, there was no "cure"; women were being treated for "vicarious menstruation." In 1844 an English gynecologist Samuel Ashwell suggested abstinence from alcohol, exercise and becoming a vegetarian would help women with this affliction. Despite his work in the area, he did not see menopause as a disease. A century later, the role of estrogen and progesterone were discovered, and hormone therapy was adopted as a form of treatment. During 1976, in Paris, France there was the first international congress for menopause held. Various countries participated and formed their national societies on menopause.

In hindsight when thinking about the women murdered for witchcraft in Salem, Massachusetts in 1962, of the 16 women killed, about 13 of them were menopausal. Could it be that they were going through menopausal symptoms, hot flashes, insomnia, and mood dysregulations and were misunderstood as participating in witchcraft?

Women are not the only ones who undergo hormonal changes as they age. In fact, men also have hormonal changes with resultant libido and testosterone level changes in middle aged men, called andropause.

THE CULTURAL PERSPECTIVE

Diversity among cultures and understanding the presentation of symptomatology and how it is perceived is very important. In the western hemisphere, women perceive menopause with a negative connotation, which is termination of childbirth, becoming old, with a less important role in society, they may or may not experience changes in their demeanor. The most common presenting symptoms include hot flashes and night sweats.

During 1970's Dr. Marcha Flint was the first anthropologist who attempted to look at menopause in non-western hemisphere, in India. She did not notice any of the menopausal symptoms that were seen in the West. In India, especially Rajasthan, women accept it with positive attributes of more privileges, more inclusive in the society, not secluded, and the most common presenting symptom being loss of vision- later found. The Mayan women also looked forward to new status and freedom (Stefanopoulou), despite experiencing uncomfortable symptoms. During 1980's Margaret Lock noted that Japanese women would present with shoulder pain and stiffness.

The difference in symptomatology experience remains an enigma, still unclear if it is due to diet, environmental factors, stress or genetic predispositions. It may be worth taking into consideration the advice from Dr. Ashwell, the gynecologist from London, who stated that exercise, abstinence from alcohol and vegetarian food may be helpful during the transition.

Physiology

Every female is born with a fixed number of eggs between one to two million immature eggs. A woman will ovulate monthly once the menstrual cycle starts. On average, 300-500 eggs will mature during a life time of ovulation. There are hormonal changes that occur prior to blood shedding and afterward that are regulated by the hypothalamic–pituitary Axis (HPA). During these hormonal changes the female body is protected from much medical comorbidity such as hypertension, strokes, osteoporosis that all surfaces once the female reaches menopause. The gonadotropin releasing hormone is released from the hypothalamus which in turn stimulates the release of follicular stimulating hormone (FSH) and luteinizing hormone (LH). They are released in blood stream and go to the endometrium, the inner layer of the uterus sloughing off, while the follicles in the ovum (the egg) prepare for ovulation in the next 10 days. Thus the inner layer sheds; hence the bleeding occurs on the first few days. While the levels of estrogen are rising in the proliferative phase of follicular cycle. Therefore, the female is more emotional and sensitive when she is bleeding and during the follicular stage. Estrogen is a hormone which relaxes the muscles, hence men have stronger muscles than women; increases the protein production in the liver, increases irritability, hence women are more sensitive during their menses; varicose veins may be more prominent due to elasticity of smooth muscles, but it protects the female from myocardial infarctions, strokes, osteoporosis. During this which the proliferative stage, the FSH increases while the LH remains in low levels, therefore the negative feedback occurs in the pituitary gland, decreasing FSH. Within the Pineal gland, which is our internal clock, it gets resets and by the day 14 there will be a peak on LH resulting in ovulation. During this time a female may feel the mittleschmerz pain, that is the pain felt during the ovulation, usually thin women are more prone to feeling the egg ovulate, i.e., out of the ten follicles only one ovulates, while the remaining die. The last stage of menstruation is the luteal phase where the progesterone dominates, which prepares the uterus for a potential fertilization, this occurs between days 15-28. During this luteal (secretory) stage, progesterone increases the appetite of the women, aggression, pica may occur, acnes on the face, melasma (grayish brownish skin discoloration), hypotension, results in dilutional anemia, etc. Keeping this in mind, when a female undergoes menopause, the above mentioned functions of hormones become dysregulated, thus affecting the biology of the woman's body, followed by her psychosocial status. The FSH to LH ratio during menopause is 3:1. Thus hot flushes, sweating, insomnia, are more prominent, along with irritability, consistent with diagnosis of menopause, after a period of 12 months of amenorrhea, the absence of menstrual cycle.

Diagnostic Criteria

To officially diagnose menopause, clinicians will take a thorough history of the menstrual cycle and check hormone levels. In menopause, there will be an increase in the follicular stimulating hormone with a decrease in estradiol.

Menopause is considered when a female ceases shedding blood for at least 12 month consecutively. Some of the medical causes that result in early onset of menopause are ovarian failure, thyroid gland disorders (hyper or hypo-functioning), medication induced menopause when giving the patient Hormone Replacement Therapy due to excessive or painful bleeding associated with endometriosis, and surgically induced menopause due to hysterectomy with or without oophorectomy (removal of the uterus with or without removal of ovaries).

Symptoms Related to Menopause

Symptoms can range from mild to moderate or severe. Literature states that the symptoms can start as early as six years prior to the onset of menopause, a state known as perimenopause. The female may present with weakness, nausea, lightheadedness, mood changes, heartburn, tachycardia, thinning of the hair, irregular weight gain, and irregular menstrual cycles. Once Menopause ensues, the female will experience more dramatic symptoms of vaginal dryness which in turn will affect her libido due to a decrease in estrogen. The decrease in estrogen can increase the risk of urinary tract infections, as the pH in the urine also changes due to changes in estrogen. A proportion of women during this time in their life will experience symptoms of depression. In some cases, the presentation will be mild and not require treatment, however, in a small percentage, the symptoms may be severe enough to warrant psychiatric evaluation. Symptoms such as worthlessness, intense dissatisfaction with one's appearance and suicidal ideation should not be minimized and these women should seek out or be referred to treatment. In other extreme circumstances, there may be an excessive preoccupation with one's appearance resulting in an uptick of cosmetic surgery at this stage of their life.

Medical risks of osteoporosis, cardiovascular symptoms, cerebrovascular symptoms increase and start to equate with that of men. During this time it is crucial that a woman has all the support she needs from her social support. This period may bring about feelings of inadequacy as a mother, spouse, daughter or friend. Irritability, short temper, throwing temper tantrums can also manifest.

How to Cope

The importance of addressing the issues at hand, having a support system, having a better understanding and self-reflection are crucial for a smoother transition into this new phase of a woman's life. Education not only for the woman experiencing the symptoms, but also for the partner and family members are necessary to ease into this new phase.

Men and Menopause?

While there is no well-defined menopausal period for men, there has been emerging literature that men may also be affected by hormonal changes. Decreases in testosterone – which may begin as early as mid-thirties, may result in changes in libido, feelings of inadequacy, fatigue and changes in mood.

Menopause and Mental Health

There is an estimate that 1.3 million women reach menopause every year in United States of America, with a prevalence of 20% report depression at some point during menopause. Such changes can overwhelm one's life, especially if not informed and unaware of what to expect. Mental wellness can be impacted as the frustration of the individual increases, resulting in increased stress thus clouding the judgement and the insight, leading to interpersonal relationship breakdowns, mood swings, impacting the self-esteem, negative thought process and behavior affecting the core believe of the individual. Other psychiatric disorders that can peak during the transition from perimenopause to menopause are Schizophrenia (only in women aged 45-50 years); panic attacks, worsening panic disorder may be more prominent among women with stressful lives, medical comorbidities with or without functional impairment. Furthermore, new onset or relapse of obsessive compulsive disorder (OCD) may be related to changes in the hormones during menopause, as well as symptoms of bipolar disorder, depressive type are more prominent during premenopausal years.

TREATMENT

Recognizing the symptoms and understanding what is going on with one's body is the most important piece when addressing menopause. There are various proposed treatments; if one had to put them in two categories then we would divide them into homeopathic/alternative and conventional medicine which can involve pharmacologic alone and or psychotherapeutic approaches.

From the homeopathic/alternative medicine review it was noted that women have used black cohosh; red clover, kava, dong quai, primrose oils, ginseng, acupuncture to address the symptoms accompanied with menopause.

FDA approved medications for menopause primarily include hormonal therapy such as Estrogen or Progesterone replacement and a combination of both Estrogen and Progesterone. There are however some absolute contraindications for hormone replacement therapy include: breast cancer, idiopathic vaginal bleeding, and liver failure. FDA approved treatments for vasomotor symptoms such as hot flashes include: Paroxetine or Brisdelle, a selective serotonin reuptake inhibitor.

Table 1. Summary of menopausal stages, symptoms and treatment

Menopausal Stages	Symptoms of Menopause	Treatment
Perimenopause: • Can occur as early as 6 years prior to menopause. Menopause: • When a female stops menstruating for 12 consecutive months. • Age of Onset: 45-55 years	• Weakness • Fatigue • Weight Gain • Mood Changes • Suicidal Thoughts • Homicidal Thoughts • Aggressive Behavior • Hot Flashes • Vaginal Dryness • Painful Intercourse • Urinary Tract Infections • Heart Palpitations • Night Sweats	• Herbal/Homeopathic Therapy • Conventional Medical Therapy • Individual Psychotherapy • Supportive Therapy

References

Baron, Y. M. (2012). A History of the Menopause. Retrieved December 05, 2018, from https://www.um.edu.mt/ms/obsgynae/research; Research - *Obstetrics & Gynaecology* p.5-6.

Butler L, Santoro N. The reproductive endocrinology of the menopausal transition. *Steroids*. 2011 Jun. 76(7):627-35.

Burt VK, Rasgon N. Special considerations in treating bipolar disorder in women. *Bipolar Disord*. 2004 Feb. 6(1):2-13.

Holesh JE, Lord M (2018). *Physiology, Ovulation. StatPerals (internet) Treasure Islan* (FL). StatPerals Publishing; 2018-2018 Oct 27. Retrieved on March 3rd, 2019 from https://www.ncbi.nlm.nih.gov/pubmed/28723025.

Marsh WK, Templeton A, Ketter TA, Rasgon NL. Increased frequency of depressive episodes during the menopausal transition in women with bipolar disorder: Preliminary Report. *Journal of Psychiatric Research*. 2008. 42:247-51.

Menopause Food and Drug Administration (n.d.). Retrieved December 05.2018 from https://www.fda.gov/menopause.

Rosenhek J (2014). *Mad with Menopause*. February 2014. Retrieved on March 3, 2019 from http://www.doctorsreview.com/history/mad-menopause/.

Singh A., Kaur S. Walia I. (2002). A historical perspective on menopause and menopausal age. *Bull Indian Inst Hist Med Hyderabad*. 2002 Jul-Dec;32(2):121-35. Retrieved March 3, 2019 from https://www.ncbi.nlm.nih.gov/pubmed/15981376.

Soares CN. Perimenopause-related mood disturbance: an update on risk factors and novel treatment strategies available. Meeting Program and Abstracts. Psychopharmacology and Reproductive *Transitions Symposium. American Psychiatric Association 157th Annual Meeting;* May 1-6, 2004; New York, NY. Arlington, Va: American Psychiatric Publishing; 2004. 51-61.

Smoller JW, Pollack MH, Wassertheil-Smoller S, Barton B, Hendrix SL, Jackson RD, et al. Prevalence and Correlates of Panic Attacks in Postmenopausal Women. *Arch Intern Med*. Sept 2003. 163:2041-47.

In: Women's Pearls
Editors: S. Fink and P. Korenis
ISBN: 978-1-53616-103-8

Chapter 9

Acculturation, Assimilation, Immigration Issues and Women's Mental Health

Mena Mirhom**, MD
Bronx-Care Health System,
Icahn School of Medicine at Mount Sinai, New York, NY, US

Introduction

Dealing with mental health can prove to be difficult, even under the most ideal circumstances. In many ways, it certainly "takes a village" to successfully treat a mental health diagnosis. However, what we find in the migrant community is that not only are the conditions less than ideal, but that they can be significant barriers that need to be navigated. Every step in the diagnostic and treatment process may take on new layers of difficulty.

Language barriers, lack of community support, can compound a diagnosis that is already complex. The impact on the individual's mental

---

* Corresponding Author's Email: MMirhom@bronxleb.org.

health care is significant. According a 2010 study, women with four socioeconomic risk factors were eleven times more likely to have postpartum depression when compared to women with no socioeconomic risk factors. This dramatic increased risk is difficult to mitigate with a varied pharmacological strategy and required a personalized as well as systemic approach to the problem at hand. Ironically, even when women have an educational advantage of having a college degree in their native country, they are more likely to be underemployed in comparison to their native-born counterparts.

According to a study in Lancet, the risk of psychiatric disorders in general is increased for migrants who are seeking refuge from war or violence. The risk of post-traumatic stress disorder in particular can be up to 10 times that of the general population. There are also well documented increased rates of depression and anxiety among this population. Being subjected to a lifetime of trauma and then forced to make an often difficult journey to a new culture with little support can be overwhelming.

In this chapter, we will discuss the nature of these challenges as well as some ways that they can be changed.

What Are the Reactions to a New Culture and Environment?

The experience of facing a new culture that is far into one's own native culture forces the individual to make a choice. In order to continue to flourish in the new society there are several options that present themselves. Separation, integration, assimilation, or acculturation are some of the possibilities of that a migrant faces when first being exposed to a new culture. Each of these possibilities may have a distinct impact on a person's mental health.

For women who are entering a new culture, separation maybe an initial response. The research is consistent that separation from others will tend to exacerbate symptoms of depression as well as other mental health disorders. This reaction of separation can sometimes be prompted by a fear of the unknown and the desire to preserve one score identity. In doing so, however, one is not able to properly engage in the new culture. From a mental health standpoint, this begins to pose a challenge to access to care, continuity of care, as well as the overall treatment outcome. The patient who takes the separation approach may have a difficult time venturing out a mental health provider. Even if they are able to do so physically, it may remain difficult to engage fully with the provider and allow them into the patient's world due to a fear of not being understood. At times, patients may seek out providers with a similar cultural background in order to mitigate this fear.

On the other hand, there may be a pressure to relinquish one's identity entirely in order to identify with the new culture. This also poses several challenges that may present themselves in mental health treatment. Such individuals may feel a sense of guilt and shame regarding their core identity and at times may also feel disingenuous. In women's mental health care specifically, it may pose a challenge to patient's accurately describing their symptoms or experiences. The patient may feel a certain pressure to present in a favorable light and therefore may over report or under report certain key symptoms that they perceive will be less culturally acceptable.

The stress and pressure associated with the acculturation process has been shown to be linked to a decrease in overall mental well-being as well as Anxiety, depression, alienation and loneliness. Therefore, we understand that this stress is a potential trigger for the development of mental health disorders.

It is also possible, although difficult, for an individual to maintain their core identity that is associated with their culture and also integrate with a new culture that they are now becoming a part of. This allows the individual to remain "themselves" while also being able to relate to those around them. This also enables the individual to be more comfortable in their own skin and be able to seek out mental health treatment and care once it is needed here.

Research has also shown that when immigrants begin with a certain set of protective factors against mental illness, those factors tend to decline over time in the new setting and ultimately result in a risk that resembles their non-migrant counterparts of the same origin. Therefore, we see that not only is the immigration process in itself stressful and potentially traumatic, but that there can also be a removal of the core protective factors that serve as a shield from the developing and progression of mental health's symptoms

Diagnostic Considerations

In a psychiatric evaluation, the objective data from the patient is most often communicated verbally, with some non-verbal elements added. Cultural dynamics often play a key role in the diagnostic interview and can pose a significant challenge in the diagnostic process, for individuals migrating from foreign countries; certain cultural beliefs that are normative may be difficult to differentiate from pathological conditions.

While it is impossible to provide a comprehensive list of cultural experiences among women coming from all over the world, there are some examples that we will highlight here to understand the nature of some cultural challenges and barriers to mental health care.

In a study conducted by the National Asian Women's Health Organization, the conflicting cultural values that impact Asian American women were highlighted. The study discussed that at times depression may be witnessed within the family, but the cultural norm reinforces silence for fear of stigma.

Another study from the Latino community shows that at times mental illness can be viewed as a sign of personal weakness rather than an illness to be treated. This perception can make it all the more difficult to discuss this topic with loved ones or even with medical providers in order to be connected to mental health care.

This is also similarly demonstrated in the African-American community. According to the office of minority mental health, although African American women have 20 percent increased chance of experiencing mental health symptoms, only 25% of the population seeks mental health care.

SPECIFIC DISORDERS

Anxiety disorders actually tend to be slightly less common in newly arrived immigrants compared to U.S. natives.

Protective factors that contribute to this decrease in the prevalence of anxiety disorders include close social contacts that shown to be associated with a decrease in anxiety symptoms. Even the perception in social support has shown beneficial effects and resulted in a reduction in psychological distress from potentially stressful events.

The prevalence of trauma among migrants is staggeringly high, at a rate of nearly 47%. Refugees in particular experience this at a rate that is nearly twice that of other migrants. Refugees can be exposed to significant physical or sexual trauma in their country of origin or throughout their migration journey.

This underscores the need for a more detailed history to be taken while interviewing patients from a migrant background. One should inquire regarding the circumstances of the migration, the pre-migration environment as well as a change in socio-economic status before and after migration.

SYSTEMATIC CHALLENGES TO WOMEN'S MENTAL HEALTH CARE

Other significant big picture challenges there are posed to women seeking mental health care involved in mental health care system itself. In the United States the system remains fragmented and largely fee for service. This model tends to result in significant out of pocket expenses and at times will limit access take care in an uneven fashion across immigration groups. This will largely vary based on socioeconomic factors, race, ethnicity, linguistic barriers as well as cultural barriers as well. This barrier is significant and is not to be understated because although it has an impact on all Americans in the health system, it tends to negatively impact migrant populations at a disproportionate rate.

The Role of Religion/Spirituality and Women's Mental Health

Religious and spiritual practices are largely viewed in the literature as protective factors in or associated with a decrease risk of depression, anxiety, substance use disorders, as well as suicide. There are over 3,000 peer reviewed studies on the impact of religion and spirituality on mental health. These practices and communities will often serve as a sanctuary or haven to migrant women with mental health difficulties who are navigating a new culture.

It is not uncommon for someone who does not speak the language and is not familiar with the culture to find common ground with people who are members of their own faith group. This can foster a sense of identity and familiarity in a new place and provide an extension of the native experience to some degree. There are also times when the religion or spiritual practice maybe a hindrance to a woman who is seeking mental health care. At times, women coming from very conservative cultural and religious backgrounds may find it very difficult to voice their concerns, emotions or symptoms to their loved ones.

Religious or spiritual involvement may also be a significant source of coping skills and coping mechanisms that they allow the individual to feel validated when confronting a new culture with conflicting beliefs. This may also be a source of support when experiencing discrimination.

In some conservative religious communities, mental health may be viewed as a lack of religious devotion or commitment period. This tends to increase the pressure, guilt, and fear associated with many mental illnesses. It serves as yet another barrier to women who are interested in mental health care. In such instances, it may be beneficial to involve the patient's spiritual leader in the treatment team. This can reinforce to the patient that their beliefs are valued and will enable the provider to approach the patient's recovery from their vantage point.

According to several studies, attendance in a religious community is often associated with decreased depression in adults, young adults as well as children. Some research attributes this to the role of a supportive community, while other research proposes the role of values that are reinforced that tend to have an impact on decreasing depression. One study found that the degree of a person's intrinsic religiosity is directly correlated to the potential recovery from depression following a physical illness. It was found that for every 10-point increase in a person's religiosity, there is a 70% increase in the rate of depression recovery rate. These findings are consistent for patients with a general belief in a transcendent being and belonging to any such community that shares their values and offer support.

SEEKING TREATMENT

Even when a woman is able to overcome the cultural stigma that is often encountered when seeking mental health treatment, a new layer of challenges begins to arise. Navigating the complex health system can be difficult to someone not familiar with the language, culture and customs of this system. It becomes significantly more challenging when one is not sure how to even begin.

LEGAL CHALLENGES

For many women migrating with their children and loved ones, immigration status may become another source fear, stress and worry. Being undocumented and facing the constant threat of deportation can further limit access to care and can make a patient more likely to have a lurking suspicion of the mental health system overall. It is not uncommon for the patient to be concerned that the medical provider will notify the department of homeland security once they discover the patient's immigration status.

For care that is not acute in nature, the patient's legal status may also impede their ability to qualify for certain insurance benefits, which would further limit their access to care and mental health providers.

For patients who are documented and are navigating the complex immigration system, this can also become a significant source of stress. The immigration process is often lengthy, complex and can be costly. For patients applying for asylum, the process can often also be re-traumatizing as they must repeat their traumatic experience in great detail on a variety of occasions and settings throughout the asylum process. This is often a significant trigger for patients and can make their symptoms of depression and post-traumatic stress disorder more pronounced.

TRAINING AND TREATMENT CONSIDERATIONS

Due to the variety of challenges that migrant women face and how they have a direct as well as an indirect impact on their mental health; it behooves the mental health provider to be familiar with them as we deliver care. Cultural sensitivity and trauma informed care become particularly important in this population of women that has been shown to be particularly vulnerable. It can be valuable to have a community ally or a lay health worker that has ties to the community and is entrenched in the cultural experience. These individuals would provide valuable insight and provide a level of support that would be critical in the long term recovery of the patient.

There is evidence for the effect that community programs that can reduce stigma and enable patients to perceive mental health care differently. When such programs begin in an environment that the patient already deems as trustworthy, such as their place of worship or community center, they are more likely to have a decreases suspicion of the mental health care that is being provided.

Psychoeducation plays an important role in the treatment of migrant women. A careful history will be instrumental in identifying potential cultural elements that are pertinent to treatment as well as potential misinformation regarding mental health care. Taking the time to explain the treatment to the patient, while validating and respecting their cultural perspective, will enable the provider to build rapport more effectively and translate to a better outcome for the patient.

Table 1. Specific elements to consider in treatment

• Immigration Status
• Trauma History Cultural Perception of Mental Health Care
• Religious and Spiritual Background
• Available Community Support

REFERENCES

Berry. Acculturation and adaptation in a new society. *International Migration*, (1992).

Fazel M1, Wheeler J, Danesh J. Prevalence of serious mental disorder in 7000 refugees resettled in western countries: a systematic review. *Lancet.* 2005 Apr 9-15;365(9467):1309-14.

Goyal D1, Gay C, Lee KA. How much does Low Socioeconomic Status Increase the Risk of Prenatal and Postpartum Depressive Symptoms in First Time Mothers? *Womens Health Issues*. 2010 Mar.

Immigration and mental health: Mexican Americans in the United States. *Harvard Review of Psychiatry*, *8*(2), 64–72.

Tobin, Carolyn L., PhD, RN, Di Napoli, Pam, PhD, RN, Tatano Beck, Cheryl, DNSc, CNM Refugee and Immigrant Women's Experience of Postpartum Depression: A Meta-Synthesis, FAAN. *Journal of transcultural nursing*, January 1, 2018.

In: Women's Pearls
Editors: S. Fink and P. Korenis

ISBN: 978-1-53616-103-8

Chapter 10

WOMEN AND SUICIDE

Darmant Bhullar*[*]*, MD and Felix Matos Padilla, MD
Bronx-Care Health System,
Icahn School of Medicine at Mount Sinai, New York, NY, US

INTRODUCTION

Suicide is a pandemic affecting all populations, despite the various cultural, economic and social differences these communities possess. The estimated annual mortality globally is 14.5 deaths per 100,000 people, which translates to approximately one death every forty seconds, with approximately 18/100,000 for males and 11/100,000 for females. Presently, deaths by suicide account for 1.5 percent of all deaths, and it is the tenth leading cause of death worldwide. In 1998, suicides represented 1.8 percent of the global burden of disease, and this is expected to increase to 2.4 percent by 2020. Some of the factors that impact suicide rates within populations are age, gender, relationship status, employment, family history of self-injurious behaviors, medical and psychiatric illnesses.

[*] Corresponding Author's E-mail: dbhullar@bronxleb.org.

Mental illnesses such as depression, substance use, anxiety, personality and psychotic disorders are prominent in those attempting suicide. In addition, seasons tend to have an effect on suicide rates, they peak in spring, especially among men, and are higher in women born during spring and early summer.

Females are more vulnerable to suicide due to psychopathology and psychosocial stressors. For instance different roles, responsibilities, status and power, are factors which interact with biological differences between the two genders, contributing to the differences in their social behaviors. Research also reflects that women make more suicide attempts, however, men are more likely to succeed with their attempts. Despite this interesting correlation, there is a lack of research studies that investigate the complex relationships between gender and suicidal behavior In order to prevent such fatal mortalities, it is imperative that social awareness regarding suicide, and mental health in general be prominent in all communities.

Sociocultural Factors

Sociocultural differences, including socioeconomic status, societal roles and responsibilities, as well as biological differences, including hormonal changes, pregnancy and menstruation, contribute to the differences in suicidal behavior between men and women. Experiences during childhood, especially physical and sexual abuse or other traumas, increase the risk of suicidal behavior during adolescence and adulthood. Sexual abuse is particularly more common in women, which increases their risk to develop psychiatric disorders including depression, post-traumatic stress disorder and borderline personality disorder. A history of childhood abuse also plays a role in the inheritance of suicidal behavior, as patients that have been sexually abused are more prone to transmit this behavior to their offspring. When it comes to ethnicity, European Americans have higher rates of suicide when compared to Hispanics and African Americans.

Psychiatric disorders increase the risks of unemployment, due to both functional decline and social stigma, which at the same time increases the rates of suicide in this population. Employment is not always a protective factor against suicide, as there are some occupations at an increased risk, including medical practitioners, especially females. Medical practitioners, including nurses and anesthetists, have access to medications and poisons that can be used to attempt suicide. Another difference can be found in the rates of suicide in different countries, with men leading in the majority of them, with the exception of China. It should also be mention that there are only a few studies focusing on suicidality in women, which could be explained by some authors as the general misconception that women attempt to commit suicide as a form of communication.

Marital Status

Over the years, multiple studies have demonstrated the protective effect of marriage on suicide. This is mainly due to the social, economic and emotional support provided, and the reduction of isolation experienced, because of the multiple opportunities for social activities and community integration. Masocco et al. (2008) showed that both Italian men and women, whether they are widowed, divorced, or separated are associated with higher risk of suicide. They found that marriage is protective, but the effect differs based on the gender. In comparison to married males, the suicide risk for widowed males increases by five-fold, and for divorced and/or separated males it increased by approximately 1.3-folds. For females, the suicide risk is twice as high in never married, and 1.7 times higher in widowed, divorced and/or separated females, compared to married females.

As marriage provides social support and economic security, married individuals tend to be happier than divorced ones. Thus, the absence of social integration, and overall increased psychological distress upon a disruption of alliance, leads to increased suicide risk. Due to the hardships endured by divorced individuals, they are more prone to developing mood and anxiety disorders, have poor social support and thus, an increase in suicide risk is noted.

Durkheim explains the correlation between divorce and suicide risk via the theory of social integration. Social integration is defined by the strength of an individual's ties to their society, and the stability of their social relations. The institution of marriage allows for increased social integration. Durkheim explains that marriage provides a greater coefficient of preservation, as it offers a sense of cohesiveness and support that is unavailable to single, divorce, or widowed individuals. Divorce disrupts this cohesion; it is an anomic condition, as it results from a sudden and unexpected change in one's social stature. Divorce reflects decreased integration, and overall a low coefficient of preservation. The loss of social support, decreased family integration, and feelings of isolation is a stressful crisis, causing severe psychological distress, and overall increasing one's suicide risk.

Similar to Durkheim, Verbrugge also explains that the social support and security provided by marriage, leads to happier individuals. The psychological, economic and social stress caused by divorce causes them to have a stronger representation in psychiatric populations. These individuals most commonly suffer from depression and upon decompensation have a higher risk of suicide, in comparison to married individuals. In turn, should married individuals be suffering from depression, their stronger support allows them to battle the illness in a healthier manner. Additionally, the Western culture has a strong cultural emphasis on achieving a successful and happy marriage. Thus, occurrence of divorce reinstates that one has failed at achieving this milestone. Self-injurious behaviors increase with a sense of failure, loss of self-esteem, and a lack of support.

However, studies have demonstrated an effect of gender on the correlation between divorce and suicide, where divorced men have a strong net effect on mortality from suicide, in comparison to women. This gender difference is explained by the different types of supportive networks developed by men and women. Women are more likely to form greater supportive social networks, which include meaningful friendships compared to men. This allows them to depend on these individuals upon resolution of a marriage. As men generally develop less meaningful and supportive networks, upon dissolution of their marriage, they are left without a healthy support system and more likely to feel isolated, depressed and thus, turn to suicide for emotional pain relief.

Literature review also reports that widowed individuals are 2.8 times more likely to die from suicide compared to married individuals. This effect is more so prominent in young or middle-aged men, in comparison to women. It is believed that this is due to the differences in which men and women react to crises and stress. Men associate widowhood with a decreased level of belongingness, whereas women do not associate marital status with belongingness as strongly, thus, it presents with greater obstacles for men. Additionally, they are required to take on new domestic roles which are not consistent with the masculine role they are raised with. The surviving spouse experiences loss, grief and loneliness, and these feelings cannot be buffered by family support. As men have less meaningful relationships outside of their marriage, it is harder for them to seek support needed through the bereavement process, and then they are more likely to feel more lonely than women. Furthermore, the additional stress of adapting to their changed role, which accompanies with their new marital status, can lead many into depression and suicidal thoughts. Sense of belonging is described as the perception of personal involvement in an environment, which allows individuals to feel that they are an integral component and valued member of that environment. Marriage tends to provide this sense of belongingness, and unfortunately widows experience a lowered sense of belongingness, which in turn has been associated with suicidal ideation.

When comparing single and married individuals, suicide risk is higher for non-married individuals less than sixty-five years, and in males more than females. Studies reflect that marital dissolution is a loss of a social bond, loss of a loved one, and loss of financial support. Single individuals are more vulnerable to feelings of depression, loneliness, and belongingness than those once married (divorced or widowed), thus increasing their baseline suicide risk. Lastly, as suicide occurs more frequently amongst single people, it indicates that marriage has a protective effect through the social and financial support it provides.

Young Marriages in Developing Nations

In contrast to the West, in developing countries like India, marriage appears to be less protective against suicide for women than men. This is most likely due to the circumstances under which these women partake in marriage, for example, arranged marriages, marriages without the woman's consent, domestic violence and young motherhood. Such stressors, in addition to lack of community and/or family support cause women to turn to suicide as the only solution to their suffering.

Domestic Violence

Domestic violence can be described as any action that directly causes physical or psychological harm and that occurs in a family environment. It is especially common towards women. Some of the risk factors that have been identified include a history of domestic violence during childhood, substance use, low socioeconomic status and lack of education. The World Health Organization (WHO) states that 8/100,000 women died by suicide in 2012. According to the same source, domestic violence is most common in family environment and one third of women are exposed to physical or sexual violence in the world. Domestic violence causes both physical and psychological consequences, including psychiatric disorders as post-traumatic stress disorder and depression, and it is well known that suicide could be seen as the only escape for these women. Revenge suicide has also been described in women without adequate support system in place while they are been abused, as they have their death as a way of forcing vengeance on the abuser.

Pathophysiology of Suicide

Past studies have suggested the involvement of neurobiological dysfunction in both, attempted and completed suicide. Post-mortem studies reveal central neurotransmission processes involved with the serotonin and noradrenaline systems are associated with suicide. Abnormalities with the serotoninergic system is associated with aggression, impulsivity, hopelessness, and impaired decision-making, all characteristics that lead to suicidal actions. Additionally, it also demonstrated that dysfunction of the hypothalamic-pituitary-adrenal axis may help predict suicide in depressed patients. As well as, low cholesterol has been associated with an increased suicide risk. Finally, genetic factors account for approximately forty-five percent of the variance in suicidal thoughts and behaviors, and thus far, tryptophan hydroxylase and serotonin transporter genes are associated and need to be studied further.

Clinical Risk Factors

Many of the people who attempt or commit suicide were previously diagnosed with a psychiatric disorder and were evaluated by a primary care physician within a month. Mood disorders (e.g., depression and bipolar disorder) and Schizophrenia are two of the most common disorders in patients that attempt suicide. The risk increases with comorbidities such as substance use disorders. The most common risk factor for suicidal behavior is depression, which is more common in women. Perhaps, due to the earlier age of presentation when compared to male. According to Oquendo et al., the most common risk factors for women were a previous attempt and its lethality, as well as fewer identified reasons for living. Other risk factors include hopelessness, chronic pain or medical comorbidities, command auditory hallucinations with suicidal content, and a poor support system. Approximately 4% of patients diagnosed with depression commit suicide, especially males who had been hospitalized for circumstances related to suicidal ideation. Approximately 15% of patients diagnosed with bipolar disorder commit suicide, which is associated with risk factors that include family history of suicide, rapid cycling, mixed affective, substance use and comorbid psychiatric disorders.

Patients with psychotic disorders, particularly schizophrenia, are at a higher risk of suicide when compared to the general population. The risk has been associated with affective symptoms such as hopelessness and depression, more than with positive psychotic features. Schizophrenic patients also have an increased risk for substance use and noncompliance with treatment, which puts them at higher risk for suicidality.

Eating disorders, including anorexia nervosa and bulimia, are more commonly seen in women. According to Lakshmi Vijayakumar, women diagnosed with anorexia nervosa have a 50-fold increased risk of suicide, which is the second leading cause of death in these patients. Bulimia also carries a risk for suicidality, with 35% of patients attempting to commit suicide according to L. Vijayakuma.

Suicide has also been associated with medical comorbidities, especially chronic or terminal disorders including cancer of the head and neck, human immunodeficiency virus/acquired immunodeficiency syndrome, multiple sclerosis and chronic pain. There are also major life events that could affect a population including natural disasters. The compromise of safety and well-being of individuals that can result in increased suicide rates.

METHODS

There are some differences between men and women when it comes to the lethality of the methods, as women usually choose less lethal methods including overdosing with pills, self-poisoning or cutting, but men usually choose firearms, jumping or hanging. The above explains the fact that women attempt to commit suicide more often than men, but the latter are more successful in their attempts. In developed countries, it is more common for women to use over the counter medications such as acetaminophen or non-steroidal anti-inflammatory drugs, as these are readily accessible, in contrast to undeveloped areas like rural Asia and India, where women use pesticides more often. In the United States, firearms are used in the majority of the suicide attempts, and the risks of suicide increases when they are kept in the house, especially unsecured.

Self-immolation is the act of committing suicide as a sacrifice, with methods that include setting oneself on fire and starvation. This is a common practice in places like Iran, India and Middle-East countries, as well as Indian women migrating to the England.

PROTECTIVE FACTORS

Marriage

Corcoran et al. (2008) discuss marriage being a strong protective factor against suicide, as rates are higher in never married, separated, divorced or widowed individuals. One Northern Ireland study revealed that only women ages 20-34 year-old who are never married are primarily at increased risk. This is mainly due to Durkeim's theory of social integration provided by marriage. It is also hypothesized that unmarried women older than 35 years are independent, have developed strong social support networks, and do not need the social and financial protection provided by marriage.

Pregnancy

One of the most documented protective factors for women is pregnancy, and rates of suicide are lower during pregnancy that when compared to non-pregnant women. It has also been reported that having children, especially taking care of them when they are dependent (less than 2 year-old) protects against suicide.

Gender

When compared to men, women are more likely to receive emotional support, as it is more socially accepted to ask for help. Supportive systems play an important role in suicide prevention, and they include family members and friends. Women are also more receptive when it comes to psychotherapy and are more willing to discuss their problems, when compared to men.

Prevention

Prevention of suicide attempts is complex and challenging. There are few suicide risk assessment tools available including the Columbia Suicide Risk Assessment, however there is no gold standard screening tool identified. During the initial evaluation, is the ideal time to obtain a comprehensive psychiatric history to cover aspects that could directly or indirectly affect the risks for suicide. Factors that should be covered include current suicidal ideation, psychiatric history, previous suicide attempts (including the lethality), and family history of suicide, physical/sexual abuse, substance use, medical comorbidities and protective factors. In patients that report suicidal ideation, the clinician must assess for a plan, intent and levels of hopelessness, as well as psychotic features including command auditory hallucinations with a suicidal content. With the above information the clinician should be able to decide whether the patient needs outpatient follow-up or inpatient admission. Level of observation in an inpatient unit, including constant 1:1 observation, should be considered for patients with an imminent risk of attempting suicide in the hospital.

Treatment modalities should also be considered after the above screening and assessment. Mood stabilizers, antidepressants and psychotherapy; most commonly cognitive behavioral therapy are used to prevent suicide in mood disorders. When treating patients with depression, the clinician should consider the increased risk of suicidal ideation when starting selective serotonin reuptake inhibitors, particularly in children and adolescents. Current recommendation is to prescribe these medications for moderately or severely depressed patients. Within the mood stabilizers, lithium has been researched to improve impulsivity and aggression, and has been shown to reduce the suicidality in patients with a mood disorder.

Psychotic disorders, especially Schizophrenia, increase the risk of suicide with poor adherence to treatment and the lack of consistent findings about the effectiveness of antipsychotics on suicidality. Clozapine has been shown to reduce suicidality in patient with Schizophrenia or Schizoaffective disorder, but the requirement of regular blood work places a barrier when it comes to compliance in these patients.

Table 1. Risk factors versus protective factors for suicidal behavior in women

Risk factors	**Protective factors**
Sociocultural • Single • Unemployed • Lack of Social Support • Occupational Access to Medication • Adolescents and Elderly *Clinical* • Bipolar Disorder • Depression • Psychotic Disorders • Borderline Personality Disorder • Post-Traumatic Stress Disorder • Substance Use Disorders • Chronic Pain or Medical Conditions • Previous Suicide Attempts • Family History of Suicide • Helplessness, Hopelessness *Trauma* • Domestic Violence • Physical and or Sexual Abuse	*Sociocultural* • Married • Employed • Social Support • Religious Beliefs Against Suicide *Clinical* • Absence of a Major Mental Illness • Good Health

REFERENCES

Behice, Han Almin., Emel, Koyuncu Kutuk., Funda, Gumustas. & Mustafa, Celik. (2016). Risk Factors for Domestic Violence in Women and Predictors of Development of Mental Disorders in These Women. *Arch Neuropsychiatry*, 2018, 55, 67–72. https://doi.org/10.29399/npa.19355.

Corcoran, P. & Nagar, A. (2009). Suicide and marital status in Northern Ireland. *Social Psychiatry and Psychiatric Epidemiology*, *45*(8), pp. 795-800.

Funda, Kavak., Ümmühan, Aktürk., Aysel, Özdemir. & Abdurrezzak, Gültekin. (2018). The relationship between domestic violence against women and suicide risk. Inonu Unıversity, Department of Nursing, Turkey. *Archives of Psychiatric Nursing*, *32*, (2018), 574–579.

Hawton, Keith. & Kees, Van Heeringen. "Suicide." *The International Handbook of Suicide and Attempted Suicide*, 1-6. doi:10.1002/9780470698976.ch.

Kposowa, A. (2000). Marital status and suicide in the National Longitudinal Mortality Study. *Journal of Epidemiology & Community Health*, *54*(4), pp. 254-261.

Kyung-Sook, W., SangSoo, S., Sangjin, S. & Young-Jeon, S. (2019). *Marital status integration and suicide: A meta-analysis and meta-regression*. [online] Econpapers.repec.org. Available at: https://econpapers.repec.org/RePEc:eee:socmed:v:197:y:2018:i:c:p:116-126.

Masocco, M., Pompili, M., Vichi, M., Vanacore, N., Lester, D. & Tatarelli, R. (2008). Suicide and Marital Status in Italy. *Psychiatric Quarterly*, *79*(4), pp. 275-285.

McLaren, S., Gomez, R., Gill, P. & Chesler, J. (2014). Marital status and suicidal ideation among Australian older adults: the mediating role of sense of belonging. *International Psychogeriatrics*, *27*(01), pp. 145-154.

Vijayakumar, Lakshmi. (2015). "Suicide in Women." *Indian Journal of Psychiatry*, *57*, no. 6, 233. doi:10.4103/0019-5545.161484.

In: Women's Pearls
Editors: S. Fink and P. Korenis
ISBN: 978-1-53616-103-8

Chapter 11

WELLNESS, BURNOUT AND WOMEN'S MENTAL HEALTH

Frozan Walyzada**, MD and Charles Odom, MD
Bronx-Care Hospital,
Icahn School of Medicine at Mount Sinai, New York, NY, US

INTRODUCTION

In hunter-gatherer societies, there tends to be a division of labor where women would have the responsibility of foraging and child-bearing whereas men would be responsible for big game hunting. The average work day is about 3-5 hours, depending on the group studied, where there is more time for leisure activities. It was not uncommon for the men to return without a successful hunt and ultimately it was what the women gathered that would feed everyone. Some would argue that women had the harder task given that they would have to provide sustenance on top of the responsibilities of motherhood each day as men that were off on the hunt. Modern society has led to changes in the division of labor, but how has

* Corresponding Author's Email: frozan.walyzada@gmail.com.

that impacted the responsibilities that women carry? Women have gone from 28.6% to 46.8% of the civilian labor force from 1948 to 2016 according to the United States Department of Labor Women's Bureau, 34.1% of active full-time physicians are women, there are 106 Women in Congress and 21 in the Senate in 2018. Women are working outside the home and then coming home to resume duties as a parent and partner, which has led to less time for leisure because her days are longer and filled with more demands and responsibilities.

BURNOUT

Burnout currently is not found in the Diagnostic and Statistical Manual of Mental Disorders (DSM), but can be found as an International Classification of Diseases (ICD) code as problems related to life management difficulties. Burnout has recently become a major concern as we are now more aware of the detrimental effects in the workplace, in one's home life and on one's health. Burnout is defined as physical or mental collapse caused by overwork or stress, others define it as exhaustion, cynicism and feelings of inadequacy. The exhaustion is further defined as feelings of being emotionally drained and physically overextended. The cynicism refers to distant and callous attitude toward one's job, being unmotivated and withdrawing from work, becoming less engaged. Lastly, feelings of inadequacy and incompetence associated with loss of self-confidence are part of lack of professional efficacy.

It is hard to recognize that one is starting to experience burnout as it has been known to occur over long periods of time. Some studies say that it can take anywhere from five to fifteen years. In order to combat burnout we must first be able to recognize it. Psychologist Herbert Freudenbergen and Gail North divided the process of burnout into twelve phases. Similar to that of the 5 stages of grief you do not have to hit each phase nor go in order and there is no timing allotted to each phase. Starting with phase one, it begins with a compulsion to prove oneself which often is described as excessive ambition. Phase two is defined by working harder, to the point that there is a notion of being irreplaceable as well. This leads to phase three where one may start to neglect ones needs whether it is sleep, nutrition, family/friends, but with the mindset that the sacrifice is necessary. In phase four, this is where one finds the displacement of conflicts. There is awareness that something is not right and it is unclear what the cause is. This leads to phase five where one has a revision of values. This is where one is seeking what is of import anymore. This can lead to denial of emerging problems and issues which is Phase six. Phase seven is withdrawal and this is one's search for any release and it is sometimes found through the use of drugs and alcohol. Phase eight is identified as obvious behavioral changes that are noticed by others and then accompanied by a feeling of emptiness and worthlessness. Depersonalization or losing contact with oneself is phase nine. Emptiness expansion is phase ten, and is defined by where one is desperately looking for activity. Phase eleven is depression and phase twelve is burnout. This is defined as a phase that one feels he is stuck in and one feels that they cannot escape their situation. This situation leads to such a helpless and hopeless state that the majority of burnout victims have suicidal ideations.

One of the biggest factors in being able to identify it is that it varies from person to person along with the fact that it can take years to manifest. Many studies indicate that those that report higher rates of burnout also report higher physical symptoms. Burnout has been associated with impaired job performance and serious health problems. Others have linked it to depressive symptoms even suicidal ideation. Burnout is not only about the "presence of negative emotions" but also about the "absence of positive ones" which is what mimics the depressive symptoms and anhedonia that are considered symptoms of depression.

Many different survey instruments have been used to study burnout including, but not limited to the Maslach Burnout Inventory, Oldenburg Inventory, Physician Work-Life Study's Single Item, and the Copenhagen Burnout Inventory (National Academy of Medicine). All of the previously mentioned surveys are self-reports and can be found online. The Maslach Burnout Inventory is recognized as one of the leading measures of burnout with the original one still available, but there are also subsections available geared specifically towards medical personnel, educators, a general one, and one for students. (Mind Garden Inc). This selection of different scales is important as the percentage of women in each field changes and it is important to have a consistent measure for each field. Currently 34.1% of active full-time physicians are women, and women continue to be the majority in educational fields in general being 98% of pre-k and Kindergarten teachers, 77.9% of elementary and middle school teachers, 46.6% of post-secondary professors, and 62.3% of educational administration, and over 50% of university students are women as per the Department of Labor Women's Bureau.

Recently there have been a number of studies looking at burnout as there has been an increase in stress-related disorders especially in service-delivery jobs such as those in the healthcare industry. Women appear to report higher levels of burnout than men in multiple studies (although one study cites that it is due to women being more likely to report it). Women cite difficulties in mastering work tasks and the demands of work-family conflict whereas their male counterparts report better work conditions and lower work-family conflicts. Other factors that impact burnout include age (more burnout at younger ages), marital status, education level of the husband and type of work of the husband (worse if the husband is in medical field), number of children (more so for children under the age of 5, but the more children, the higher risk of burnout), type of work (if there is room for growth vs a long-term more stagnant position where growth is limited), professional experience, type of shift work. "70% of Women with children under the age of 18 participate in the labor force."

Bye et al, looked at medical students that became parents during medical school, especially women, as women currently make up almost half of the medical student population in America. "Women physicians have a higher frequency of burnout (55%) than male physicians (46%)." Parenthood is stressful on its own but there is also the added stress of pregnancy, any complications and fertility issues that also add to stress leading to burnout. Due to the stress of schooling and threat of delaying graduation 72% of women stated they would have extended their maternity leave if possible. Also it was found that 32% of the pregnancies had by medical students had complications compared to the 1% that is in the general population.

Women in Medicine have a difficult task of trying to decide when or if they will have children due to the bulk of training and beginning of their career is during their mid 20's to 30's. There is a high demand for performance during this time as well, as a financial constraint due to being in school or being paid the wage of a resident/fellow. They are also faced with pursuing specialties that may offer better schedules to help with the balance of work and family. The question of when is it a good time arises, and many women recommend that to wait until after they have finished their training, but then this increases the risk for infertility and congenital abnormalities. A consensus of when it is the least favorable time to get pregnant is during the third year of medical school and during one's internship year as these are some of the most stressful times in training and the most increased chance of burnout. The timing of pregnancy is also stressed by the intensity of the training as there are some training programs that do not offer any maternity leave and female residents will have to use all their vacation time.

Although there have been changes due to the increasing number of women enrolled in medical school and becoming licensed physicians, women in medicine attempt a work life balance as they outnumber men in primary care and psychiatry, and stay away from more stressing fields of medicine such as the demands that are required like in the surgical fields except in Obstetrics and Gynocology where women are the majority Swinder et al. categorized the reasons for burnout into three categories; organizational, occupational, and individual. When looking at the stressors at the organizational level, the psychological environment was looked at in regards to the depletion of resources and the constant or increasing demands to perform. Interactions with the clients are what constitutes the occupational category and for individual they look to personality characteristics which they also cite as being the weakest indication for burnout. They do find that neurotic individuals (those that are anxious, insecure, depressed, fearful, and nervous) would be more prone to being unable to adapt to changes in their environment in comparison to someone that is more stable.

Bakker et al. looked at social workers over the course of their 3-year-study. There were reports of sleep disturbances, headaches, respiratory infections, and gastrointestinal infections. They also divided burnout to be the result of either situational factors and/or individual factors. Situational factors are job demands vs. resources that are available. The sustained effort required to meet the job demands.

Individual factors are influenced by socioeconomic status and personality variables that can be used to determine predisposing factors for burnout. Strain can be induced when personality doesn't align with the tasks given for example placing an introvert into a leadership role. Anxiety was seen to exacerbate these feelings. Similarly reported by Danhof-Pont et al, that those that were experiencing burnout had an increased incidence of common cold, flu-like illness, and gastroenteritis.

There are even biological markers that are affected when there is increased stress. It was found that blood work from those that were identified as experiencing burnout had low levels of prolactin, which is not often a concern but can have an effect on reproduction. They were also found to have higher levels of TNF-α, an immune marker that is part of the inflammatory process that takes place in the acute phase of an infection. They were also found to have higher Hemoglobin A1C, a unit that measures the function of insulin and can be used to indicate insulin resistance syndrome (IRS), characterized by hyperinsulinemia, hyperglycemia, hypertension, dyslipidemia, and abdominal obesity. Ironically in men it was found that burnout would cause higher levels of prolactin.

PREVENTING BURNOUT

It has been found that there are ways to buffer stressors with positive coping resources and having a positive support system. It was also shown that having a recovery period would lead to better work engagement which would then lead to better life satisfaction. It is also noted that it is not the quantity of work/stress because "If someone works 12 hours a day, every day, yet still has found a way to relax, he will very likely have no problem." "On the other hand, someone else may find a part-time job extremely stressful and develop burnout syndrome." -Staedt

Making recovery a priority over the weekend and in the evenings is important for general well-being and performance. Danhof-Pont et al. list that with psychological treatment, consisting of relaxation therapy, cognitive therapy, learning of coping skills, and reactivation, can reduce complaints effectively. One article defined the way of preventing burnout is following two rules. First is to "budget your physical resources" which included enough sleep, wholesome food, and regular exercise. Rule number two was to aim for equilibrium between tension and relaxation. This means to have your personal stress reducer whether it is exercising, watching TV, listening to music, or your hobby, because if you reduce your stress level the work you need to get done won't be as daunting as it used to be. In addition to the two rules it recommended to be social, and be in contact with friends and family as well as learning relaxation techniques like yoga, or progressive muscle relaxation. This all leads back to the importance of leisure time providing women an opportunity to recover in an effort to prevent burnout. One author looked at burnout after not taking a day off for five years and stated there are four things you can do to prevent and get yourself out of burn out. First is to have discipline, to get up and do what must be done as this gives a sense of purpose in life and work. Second is breaking down tasks to smaller more manageable "chunks" that will be realistically able to be done. Third is taking time off of social media as it takes away productive time and subliminally you end up focusing on a possible false reality which is portrayed on the internet where "the truth is almost certainly most aspect of their lives suck." Fourth is exercise where you focus on pushing yourself for a short period of time, and not taking leisure walks as this isn't working out.

Table 1. Definition of Burnout

Signs and Symptoms • Stages of Burnout • Physical symptoms • Burnout scales • Factors that contribute to burnout • Burnout and pregnancy complications • Burnout and family planning • Physical symptoms of burnout • Biomarkers
Prevention and Recovery • relaxation therapy • cognitive therapy • learning of coping skills • Reactivation • Physical resources (enough sleep, wholesome food, and regular exercise) • Personal stress reducers (watching TV, listening to music, or your hobby) • Contact with Friends and family • Leisure activities

REFERENCES

Bakker, Arnold and Costa, Patricia, "Chronic job burnout and daily functioning: A theoretical analysis" *Burnout Research,* no 1 (April 2014):112-119.

Bianchi, R. et al. "Biological research on burnout-depression overlap: Long-standing limitations and on-going reflections" *Neuroscience and Biobehavioral reviews,* no 83 (October 2017): 238-239.

Bianchi, R. et al. "Burnout-depression overlap: A review" *Clinical Psychology Review,* no 36 (January 2015): 28-41.

Bye, E, et al. "Pregnancy and Parenthood during Medical School South Dakota Medicine" *South Dakota Medicine* 70, no12 (December 2017): p551-555.

Danhof-Pont, Marie Bernadine; et al. Biomarkers in burnout: A systematic review" *Journal of Psychosomatic research,* no 70 (October 2010): 505-524.

Dyrbye, L. et al. "Association of Clinical Specialty with Symptoms of Burnout and Career Choice Regret Among US Resident Physicians" *JAMA 320*. no 11 (September 2018): 1114-1130.

Ellison, K. "Severe Complications for Women during Childbirth Are Skyrocketing — and Could Often Be Prevented" *ProPublica* Dec. 22, 2017, 5 a.m. EST.

Grossi, G. et al. "Physiological correlates of burnout among women" *Journal of Psychosomatic Research*, no 55 (September 2002): 309-316.

Khosravi, S. et al. "Estimation of burnout status of women employees of health centers of Tehran city community" *Nursing Practice Today, no* 5 (March 2018): 290-98.

Kraft, U. "Burned out Your job is extremely fulfilling. It is also extremely demanding--and you feel overwhelmed. You are not alone" *Scientific American Mind* (2006).

Lennartsson, AK, H Billig, IH Jonsdottir, "Burnout is Associated with Elevated Prolactin Levels in Men but not in Women" *Journal of Psychosomatic Research* 76, no 5 (May 2014): 380-383.

Shukla, R. *12 Stages of Burnout and 4 things you can do about it! Success and Happiness*, Wednesday, 10/4/2017 Retrieved 12/5/18.

Swider Brian and Ryan Zimmerman, "Born to Burnout: A meta-analytic path model of personality, job burnout, and work outcomes" *Journal of Vocational Behavior,* no 76 (December 2010): 487-506.

Upadyaya, K. et al. "From job demands and resources to work engagement, burnout, life satisfaction, depressive symptoms, and occupational health" *Burnout Research*, no 3(October 2016):101- 108.

Verlander, G. "Female Physicians: Balancing Career and Family" *Academic Psychiatry* 28, no 4 (Winter 2004) 331-332.

In: Women's Pearls
Editors: S. Fink and P. Korenis
ISBN: 978-1-53616-103-8

Chapter 12

THE LEGAL SYSTEM AND WOMEN'S MENTAL HEALTH

Paulina Riess*[*]*, MD
Bronx-Care Health System,
Icahn School of Medicine at Mount Sinai, New York, NY, US

INTRODUCTION

Historically the female role in society has been shaped within a patriarchal framework. Women's role in society has evolved from antiquity, through the women's right's movement of the nineteenth century up to the modern era. A multitude of issues including, but not limited to education, the right to vote, and reproductive rights have been brought to the forefront. Despite historically, and perhaps biologically having been placed in a maternal, nurturing role, women have been part of the legal system since its advent in ancient civilization. Hammurabi's Code, the first attestation of written law in eighteenth century Babylon BCE, based the magnitude of punishment contingent upon the nature of the crime

[*] Corresponding Author's E-mail: PRIESS@bronxleb.org.

committed. Gender was also taken into account as women were, for the most part, considered to be part of the lower framework of society. This is not to say that throughout history, the conviction of heinous crimes has been limited to men. One can examine cases such as Clementine Barnabet and Elizabeth Bathory to see that the female sex is quite capable of crimes as horrific as serial murder whether by axe or by iron maiden. On the other hand, one may be inclined to question how many crimes committed by women followed by punishment appropriate during the given time period have been direct sequelae of untreated mental illness or trauma? Roslyn Muraskin, has boldly stated that mentally ill female offenders have been misunderstood, feared, and stigmatized by bearing the additional stigma of a criminal label (Gido & Dalley, 2011). In their book, *Women's Mental Health Issues Across the Ciminal Justice System*, authors state that there are serious repercussions following the lack of interest, care, and treatment of mentally ill female offenders (Gido & Dalley, 2011). Unfortunately, mentally ill female offenders often face a response from the criminal justice system that more often than not, prevents these individuals from reentering society as productive citizens (Gido & Dalley, 2011). In this chapter, we examine scholarly work as it pertains to the role of mentally ill women in the criminal justice system.

WOMEN AND INCARCERATION

The number of women imprisoned in the United States has doubled in the last thirty years (Covington & Bloom, 2003). This includes confinement to state and federal prisons as well as local jails. More than one million women are currently under the supervision of the criminal justice system (Covington & Boom, 2003). Nearly three quarters of the female incarcerated population has an ongoing mental health problem with eighty percent of incarcerated women meeting criteria for at least one lifetime psychiatric disorder (Boom & Covington, 2008). Women entering the correctional system seem to be at higher risk for substance use disorders, mental illness, as well as having significant trauma history (Gido

& Dalley, 2011). In fact, the three most common diagnoses for female prisoners include substance use disorders, post-traumatic stress disorder, and depression (Boom & Covinton, 2008).

In comparison with the incarcerated male population, a smaller number of women have been incarcerated for a violent offense (Boom & Covinton, 2008). Authors of several studies reiterate that most violent crimes committed by women have been in the context of extreme physical or sexual abuse emphasizing that the incarcerated woman is more likely to report a history of physical, sexual, or emotional abuse (Bloom & Covinton, 2008). Girls and women experience more frequent and more serious victimization than boys and men with women being more likely to react to victimization with depression (Boom & Covinton, 2008). Judith Herman offers a three state model for providing trauma services to women which encompasses educating women as to what trauma and abuse are, validating their reactions, and providing coping skills (Gido & Dalley, 2011). Despite societal progress with advocacy pertaining to women's rights, scholarly work continues to point out that women continue to be at the social and economic margins of society rendering them at greater risk for domestic violence and sexual assault. Women's status remains low worldwide with low status itself being a mental health risk (Afifi, 2007).

Mental Health Treatment While Incarcerated

The treatment strategy pertaining to the mentally ill population within the criminal justice system cannot have a gender neutral approach. Based on the information available, a gender responsive approach is crucial when addressing the mental health needs of these women (Afifi, 2007). In the article titled *Gender Differences in Mental Health.* Authors identify the need to develop mechanisms to monitor gender sensitivity in the mental health system. Undoubtedly, this extends to the criminal justice system. The foundation seems to lie in strengthening community services and increasing public awareness in order to decrease stigma associated with mental illness. A femicentric approach is one particular model that would encompass gender sensitive services for mentally ill women in the mental health court system (Gido & Dalley, 2011). Such an approach could integrate a female based perspective and female based analysis into understanding the problems of women in society as a whole.

NATURE OF CRIMES PERTAINING TO WOMEN

Acts of criminal violence are generally thought of as pertaining to men. In their paper titled *Female Crimes of Violence*, Rosenblatt and Greenland argue that there have been quantitative differences in the criminal behavior of men and women (Rosenblatt & Greenland, 1974). In lieu of growing liberties granted to women along with a societal shift in the western world equalizing the sexes, these authors state that the rate of violent crimes committed by women has been increasing since 1969. A more recent statistical analysis shows that between 1990 and 1998, the number of female defendants convicted of felonies in State courts grew at more than twice the rate of increase for male defendants (Greenfeld & Snell, 1999). In their paper *Female sex offenders: Clinical and demographic features* Nathan and Ward found that rejection and revenge played a role in female sex offenders who served as accomplices to men (Nathan & Ward, 2002). O'Connor provided the following statistics in his paper titled *Female sex offenders: Information on 19 women convicted of indecency and 62 women convicted of other sex offences was examined. Those convicted of indecency offences often had poor social skills and had a high incidence of mental illness, mental handicap and alcoholism. Two were convicted of indecent exposure, a rare offence in women. In 39 (63%) of the sex offences with individual victims, the victims were children and in 9 cases the offender was the mother or step-mother. In 25 cases the women were convicted of aiding and abetting a male offender. Of those convicted of indecent assault on persons under 16 and of gross indecency with children, 48% had a previous history of psychiatric disorder* (O'Connor, 2002). Hence, literature points to violent crimes including but not limited to murder, assault, and sexual offenses as not being exclusive to the male perpetrator.

Table 1. Mechanisms to monitor gender sensitivity in the mental health and criminal justice system

1. Strengthening community services.
2. Increasing public awareness including public and government policy makers.
3. Decreasing stigma associated with mental illness.
4. Implementing a gender responsive (femicentric) approach when addressing the mental health needs of women.

Mental Illness as It Relates to Women Who Commit Crimes, Return to the Community, and Recidivism

In their systematic study focusing on incarcerated women, Cloninger and Guze stated that all the female offenders had at least one psychiatric diagnosis (Cloninger & Guze, 2006). The diagnoses in this particular population mostly included personality disorders and substance use disorders (Cloninger & Guze, 2006). In their paper titled *Mentally disordered women in jail: who receives services?* Teplin, Abram, and Mclelland make clear two pertinent findings. The first is that many jail inmates carry diagnoses of mental disorders and require treatment (Teplin, Abram, Mclelland, 1997). The second being that less than one quarter of female jail detainees who had severe mental disorders and needed service received them while incarcerated. Gido and Dalley dedicated an entire chapter to this topic titled, *Women Destined to Failure: Policy Implications of the Lack of Proper Mental Health and Addiction Treatment for Female Offenders*. The authors state that the data clearly shows that women need addiction and mental health treatment before, during, and after imprisonment. They conclude by stating that the rate of recidivism is contingent upon the treatment that prisoners receive (Gido & Dalley,

2011). The authors of this book also emphasize that effective prison based programming for women is *key* for women with serious mental illness (Gido & Dalley, 2011). They state the following: *These provisions must look beyond core legal requirements and gender neutral service standards and toward the specific needs of incarcerated women both in prison and upon their eventual return to the community* (Gido & Dalley, 2011). Literature points to a vast number of female prisoners having a history of mental illness. In conclusion, it is imperative to address the need for treatment in order to reduce the rate of recidivism.

PREGNANCY

The topic of pregnancy within the incarcerated population has been prevalent throughout history, and continues to be an important factor addressed by the modern prison system. Daniel Defoe became fascinated with a female prisoner by the name of Moll King whom he met during a visit to London's Newgate Prison. He partially based his 1722 novel Moll Flanders on their conversations. Fictional Moll led a life of thievery, prostitution, and scandal. One pertinent fact in her life story is that is that she was the daughter of a convicted felon, having been born in Newgate Prison. Moll's mother "pleaded her belly" and was offered a stay of execution (Defoe, 1722). One can't help, but speculate whether Moll's life would have taken a different turn had if her mother had access to a program which took into account maternal infant needs. In her paper titled Perinatal needs of Pregnant, Incarcerated Women, Hotelling states that pregnant prisoners have health care needs that are not adequately met by the prison system (Hotelling, 2008). The author continues by emphasizing that many of these women have high risk pregnancies due to a low socioeconomic background (Hotelling, 2008). Siefert and Pimlott argue that studies of pregnancy outcome among prisoners demonstrate high rates of perinatal mortality and morbidity (Siefert & Pimlott, 2001). The authors emphasize that innovative residential programs for drug dependent pregnant prisoners may improve overall pregnancy outcome. Cassidy states that pregnant female offenders face multiple adversities that make successful parenting difficult resulting in their children being at risk of developing insecure attachment (Cassidy et al., 2009). The authors concluded their study by emphasizing the following: "In the present study, following intervention in a jail-diversion program, we found rates of infant attachment security and disorganization equivalent to those typical of low-risk samples, and found that the mothers in our study were as sensitive as mothers in an existing community sample. These results are striking given the multirisk nature of our sample" (Cassidy et al., 2009). In conclusion literature emphasizes the importance of adequate treatment as well as access to resources including programs for the incarcerated, pregnant population. Such programs either in the prison system or through court diversion seem to benefit both mothers and their infants in the long run.

CONCLUSION

I would like to conclude this chapter by stating that literature regarding incarcerated women points to three pertinent areas. The first being that an abundance of incarcerated women suffer from mental illness diagnoses and are in dire need of adequate treatment. Secondly, rates of recidivism have been proven to decrease if access to treatment encompassing appropriate programs is readily available to female convicts. Lastly, a femicentric approach to the treatment of incarcerated women has been shown to be an effective tool in maintaining wellbeing and decreasing rates of recidivism.

Table 2. Conclusive Findings

1. Incarcerated women suffer from mental illness and require treatment.
2. Access to sufficient treatment decreases rates of recidivism.
3. A femicentric approach to treatment has been shown to be an effective tool in decreasing rates of recidivism.
4. Programs for pregnant, incarcerated prisoners benefit mothers and infants in the long term.

References

Afifi, M. (2007). Gender differences in mental health. *Singapore medical journal*, *48*(5), 385.

Bloom, B. E. & Covington, S. (2008). Addressing the mental health needs of women offenders. *Women's mental health issues across the criminal justice system*, 160-176.

Cassidy, J., Ziv, Y., Stupica, B., Sherman, L. J., Butler, H., Karfgin, A. & & Powell, B. (2010). Enhancing attachment security in the infants of women in a jail-diversion program. *Attachment & Human Development*, *12*(4), 333-353.

Cloninger, C. R. & Guze, S. B. (1970). Psychiatric illness and female criminality: The role of sociopathy and hysteria in the antisocial woman. *American Journal of Psychiatry*, *127*(3), 303-311.

Covington, S. & Bloom, B. E. (2003). Gendered justice: Women in the criminal justice system. *Gendered justice: Addressing female offenders*, 3-23.

Defoe, D. (2005). Moll Flanders. Broadview Press.

Gido, R. L. & Dalley, L. (2011). Women's mental health issues across the criminal justice system. Pearson Higher Ed.

Greenfeld, L. A. & Snell, T. L. (1999). Women offenders (p. 1). Washington, DC: US Department of Justice, Office of Justice Programs, Bureau of Justice Statistics.

Hotelling, B. A. (2008). Perinatal needs of pregnant, incarcerated women. *The Journal of perinatal education*, *17*(2), 37.

McClellan, D. S., Farabee, D. & Crouch, B. M. (1997). Early victimization, drug use, and criminality: A comparison of male and female prisoners. *Criminal justice and behavior*, *24*(4), 455-476.

Nathan, P. & Ward, T. (2002). Female sex offenders: Clinical and demographic features. *Journal of Sexual Aggression*, *8*(1), 5-21.

O'Connor, A. A. (1987). Female sex offenders. *The British Journal of Psychiatry*, *150*(5), 615-620.

Rosenblatt, E. & Greenland, C. (1974). Female crimes of violence. *Canadian J. Criminology & Corrections*, *16*, 173.

Siefert, K. & Pimlott, S. (2001). Improving pregnancy outcome during imprisonment: a model residential care program. *Social Work*, *46*(2), 125-134.

Teplin, L. A., Abram, K. M. & McClelland, G. M. (1997). Mentally disordered women in jail: Who receives services? *American Journal of Public Health*, *87*(4), 604-609.

https://www.nami.org/Learn-More/Public-Policy/Jailing-People-with-Mental-Illness, retrieved 2/1/19.

In: Women's Pearls
Editors: S. Fink and P. Korenis

ISBN: 978-1-53616-103-8

Chapter 13

SUBSTANCE USE DISORDER AND WOMEN'S MENTAL HEALTH

***Pankaj Manocha, MD*[1], *Jayanta Chowdhury**, *MD*[1] *and Sabina Fink, MD*[1,2]**

[1]Bronx-Care Hospital, Icahn School of Medicine at Mount Sinai, New York, NY, US
[2]Northwell Health, Garden City Treatment Center, Garden City, NY, US

INTRODUCTION

Traditionally there have been higher rates of substance use among men when compared to women. However, the recent surveys have showed that this gap between men and women have reduced over the last 2 decades. As per National Institute of Drug Abuse 2017 report, although men are more likely to die due to a drug overdose; women are more susceptible to craving and relapse in the substance use cycle. Studies on gender difference and substance use have shown that there is an accelerated

* Corresponding Author's E-mail: JChowdhu@bronxleb.org.

progression of development of substance use disorder among women when compared to men for opioids, cannabis, and alcohol. This phenomenon of accelerated progression from the time they start using substances, to the onset of dependence and seeking treatment is termed as Telescoping.

Opioid Epidemic

Opioid use has been a major challenge over the past decade among the United States health care practitioners. As per fact sheet released from White House, the current administration had awarded over six billion dollars to be work against the opioid epidemic. President Trump's administration initiative includes providing education on ill effects of drugs; reduce the flow of drugs in communities and across the United States borders and funding the research by expanding evidence-based treatments for opioid addiction. Of the money allocated above one billion dollars were awarded to state and local agencies to address the opioid crisis.

Current Opioid Crisis; Statistics of Females vs. Males

Opioids were the most common contributor to overdose related deaths in Caucasian men, Caucasian women and Hispanic women. Heroin was the most common contributor to overdose related deaths in Hispanic men. There has been a recent steep increase in drug overdose death for African American and Hispanic men and women secondary to heroin per Center for Disease Control (CDC), 2017 report.

Prescription Opioids

A meta-analysis published showed that women are more sensitive to pain and more likely to have chronic pain when compared to men, hence have high rates of opioid prescriptions in reproductive age women. There is also evidence in literature, which shows that women had significantly higher likelihood of self-medicating with pain medications for stress and anxiety. Therefor may result in a lethal overdose, which occurs as opioids suppress breathing. As per CDC data from 1999 to 2016, deaths from prescription opioid overdoses increased more rapidly for women (596 percent or sevenfold) than for men (312 percent or fourfold). The age group of women, which is affected the most and more likely to die from a prescription opioid overdose, is between 45 to 54 years (CDC, 2017). Heroin deaths among women increased at more than twice the rate than compare to men from 1995-2016. There is a steep increase in the rates of synthetic opioid-related deaths among women by 850 percent between 1999 and 2015 (CDC, 2017).

HEROIN AND INTRAVENOUS DRUG ABUSE

As per current literature women are more likely to use injection of drugs if their sexual partners are injecting heroin. Women are also more likely than men to be introduced to injection by their sexual partners. One of the studies showed that 51% of the female heroin users were first injected by their male sexual partner, on the contrary; with men, a friend injected 90% of first time use.

MATERNAL OPIOID TREATMENT: HUMAN EXPERIMENTAL RESEARCH (MOTHER) STUDY

MOTHER study is sentinel study highlighting the treatment options (methadone or buprenorphine) for opioid dependent pregnant women. Subjects were 175 pregnant opioid dependent women whom were randomized into two groups buprenorphine vs. methadone. Neonates of the women (58 buprenorphine & 73 to methadone = 113) were followed. Study showed that buprenorphine exposed infants required 89% less morphine, 43% fewer hospital days, & 58% shorter duration of treatment for the neonatal opioid withdrawal syndrome (NAS). There was more maternal drop-out in buprenorphine vs. methadone group (33% vs. 18%) and this dropout is proposed to be due to induction protocol at least in part, as per research.

Prescription Opioid Addiction Treatment (POATS) Study

POATS is National Institute of Drug Abuse funded clinical trial (N=653; 40% women), where investigators did not find any gender difference in opioid dependence severity or treatment outcomes. However, it was highlighted that women had greater functional impairment, psychiatric severity, and are more likely to use prescription opioids to cope with negative affect and pain; on the other hand, men had more opioid craving and significant alcohol use than women.

Opioid Use Disorder and Psychiatric Disorders

The Co-occurrence of psychiatric disorders is under-recognized in Opioid Use Disorder (OUD), but is an important consideration not only for understanding the OUD, but also for better understanding of treatment outcomes. The data shows that individuals with psychiatric diagnosis are more likely to misuse prescription pain medications. On comparison, individuals misusing opioids with no mental illness (3.3%) is far less than individuals in any mental illness which is accounted for 11.1% of serious persistent mental illness. Individuals with OUD are at increased risk for psychiatric disorders such as Anxiety, Depression, and Post Traumatic Stress Disorder. In Individuals with OUD, the lifetime prevalence of mood disorder is 54%, anxiety disorder is 36% and these individuals with OUD are five times more likely to develop mood disorder and three times more likely to develop anxiety disorder when compared to other individuals. In individuals with OUD there is a high risk of completed suicide, which is more prevalent in men then women; however there is a significantly elevated risk in women with OUD for chronic pain, depression and anxiety.

MEDICATION ASSISTED TREATMENT (MAT)

MAT at present is the treatment of choice for OUD patients. This treatment includes medications combined with behavioral counseling for a "whole patient" approach. Medications, including buprenorphine, methadone, and extended release intramuscular naltrexone are effective for the treatment of opioid use disorders. A study conducted by National Institute on Drug Abuse (NIDA) showed similar results once treatment is initiated. Either buprenorphine/naloxone combination or extended release naltrexone formulation are similarly effective in treating opioid use disorder. However, intramuscular naltrexone requires several steps prior to administration. First, evaluation of the Liver Function, followed by opioid detoxification, lastly prior to intramuscular monthly injection an oral naltrexone challenge. The oral challenge is to evaluate the reaction, potential side effect to the medication prior to long acting intramuscular injection. Once detoxification was complete, both medications had similar effectiveness.

Buprenorphine and methadone are most commonly prescribed MAT. In controlled environment either methadone treatment clinic, or outpatient treatment clinics, both successfully assist in the treatment of opioid use disorder. In one of the recent meta-analysis it was shown that methadone treatment has some advantage and is associated with higher treatment retention.

Substance Use While Pregnant and Breastfeeding

There is substantial evidence in literature that supports the dangerousness of substance use to an unborn child. The use of tobacco, consumption of ethanol, or any other illicit drug use during pregnancy or during lactation period may have severe consequences on the fetus. The risk is doubled for stillbirth as compared to non-drug user. The risk of stillbirth from tobacco use is 2.8 folds higher among daily smokers, followed by cannabis, and prescription strength pain medication which increasing stillbirth to 2.3 folds. Passive transport or second hand smoke exposure with tobacco also doubles the risk of stillborn. These substances are known to easily transfer through placenta to fetus or through breast milk to the newborn. It is estimated that about 5 percent of pregnant women use one or more addictive substances.

Neonatal Abstinence Syndrome (NAS)

As per the data from NIDA, NAS has increased nearly fivefold nationally the years between 2000 to 2012. The severity of withdrawal depends on several factors, including the length and duration of use. Another key factor is, whether the newborn is full term or premature, plays a significant role. Full term NAS severity is slightly less. The signs and symptoms of newborn withdrawal can occur up to 2 weeks following delivery. The signs may include, but not limited to short terms effects such as fever, irritability, seizure, diarrhea, hypo or hyperactive muscle tone, trembling, sweating, and blotchy skin coloring. Some of the effects are long term and can present as birth defects, low birth weight, premature birth, small head circumference and even sudden infant death syndrome.

Substance Use Disorder Treatment for Pregnant or Lactating Mothers

As per U.S. federal law, pregnant women are entitled to priority admission into publicly funded substance use disorder treatment programs. This is to prevent the waiting times and get an instant bed in a residential program. The primary treatment provider must secure prenatal care if a pregnant woman is not already receiving such care. The studies have shown that when compared to untreated pregnant women, women treated with methadone or buprenorphine have lower risk of NAS, less severe NAS, and shorter treatment time. The neonates have older gestational age, higher weight, and closer to normal range head circumference at birth. Data shows that intensive outpatient treatment programs, which provide higher level of care than that of traditional outpatient programs, have shown better results. Data also shows that these programs tend to be more successful when they have inbuilt childcare, parenting classes and vocational training.

Treating Pregnant Women with Opioid Use Disorder

There is no U.S. Food and Drug Administration approved medications to treat opioid-dependent pregnant women. Methadone therapy or buprenorphine maintenance combined with prenatal care and a comprehensive drug treatment program is the gold standard. However, buprenorphine treatment is considered to have lower NAS. When buprenorphine was compared to methadone, it resulted in 10 percent lower incidence of NAS. Decreased neonatal treatment time by 8.46 day and less morphine needed for NAS treatment by 3.6 mg. Current guidelines recommend buprenorphine alone as treatment of choice as oppose to the combination of buprenorphine/naloxone. This however increases risk for overdose if injected, and or diversion. Methadone must also be closely monitored for Qtc prolongation, and may require split dosage, which may as well lead to diversion risk. As always a clinician must assess on case by case bases. Travel hardship may also be taken into account for those enrolled in methadone clinics, requiring six days a week pick up privileges. Coordination of care and frequent follow ups with the obstetric high risk clinic is essential for mother and the baby.

Treating of Neonates with Neonatal Abstinence Syndrome Secondary to Opioid

The treatment of the neonates may require use of methadone, morphine or buprenorphine in a hospital setting. It has been published by a NIDA-funded study that sublingual buprenorphine may have some advantage over tablet form as it resulted in shorter duration of treatment and shorted length of stay for the patient.

Alcohol Use Disorder in Women

Excessive alcohol use has led to approximately 88,000 deaths and 2.5 million years of potential life lost (YPLL) each year in the United States from years 2006 to 2010. The economic costs of excessive alcohol consumption in 2010 were estimated at $249 billion. Men are historically more likely to drink alcohol, but recently several large epidemiological studies have showed that the gender gap has been decreasing over time. According to Center for Disease Control, approximately 46% of adult women report drinking alcohol in the last 30 days, and approximately 12% of adult women report binge drinking 3 times a month. Due to gender differences in body structure and physiology women tend to absorb alcohol more rapidly, metabolize slowly hence causing higher alcohol levels in their blood than men.

Comorbid Conditions Associated with Alcohol Use Disorder: Psychiatric

Some psychiatric disorder which are associated with comorbid ethanol use are: Post-Traumatic Stress Disorder, Major Depression Disorder, Anxiety Disorder, Cognitive Impairment, Increased Suicide Risk, Decreased Rapid Eye Movement Sleep.

Comorbid Conditions Associated with Alcohol Use Disorder: Medical

Some medical diagnoses which are associated with comorbid ethanol use are: Hypertension, Fatty Liver Change, Gastro Intestinal Disturbances, Irregular Menstrual Cycle, Cardiomyopathy, Wernicke-Korsakoff Syndrome, Cerebral Atrophy, Fetal Alcohol Syndrome.

Treatment Options after Alcohol Use Disorder Is Diagnosed

Recommendation for treatment are: Intervention, Motivation (to motivate for treatment and maintain sobriety), possible involvement of family members or other social support. Detoxification-medically supervised or medically management setting are ideal. Outpatient detoxification can be challenging and dangerous, if taper of medication is not followed appropriately. Rehabilitation once medically stable and out of the danger zone of withdrawal seizures or delirium tremens. Both inpatient and outpatient rehabilitation is appropriate. Community meeting such as Alcoholics Anonymous (AA) are available in most areas, throughout the day.

Pharmacotherapy in Intoxication and Withdrawal

Patients should be monitored carefully and closely to prevent progression to alcohol withdrawal delirium (most severe form is Delirium Tremens) which is classified as shaking, rapid onset of confusion, high blood pressure, fever, and hallucinations. Usually requires an admission to the intensive care unit (ICU). Some frequently used medications: Chlordiazepoxide, Diazepam, Lorazepam, and Phenobarbital.

Rehabilitation

Several key components include: maintain motivation for abstinence, help patients readjust to lifestyle modifications, prevention of relapse. Medications used as maintenance may include: Disulfiram, Naltrexone, Acamprosate.

Gender Specific Treatment

Women are less likely to seek treatment than men, because of greater social stigma and some other socioeconomic factors such as pregnancy, child care, and concerns about child custody issues. Several studies have shown that gender specific treatment may provide a safer environment. Specifically where women with a history of trauma might not feel comfortable discussing issues related to their alcohol problems. Outpatient programs generally have gender specific groups available. These programs are more likely to address women's needs for on-site child care, prenatal care, medical and mental health providers. Such options might be available on site in some programs. These program graduation rates are expected to be higher when compared with traditional programs.

Cannabis and Women's Health

Cannabis is the most commonly used illicit drug in the United States with approximately 22.2 million users each month. Compared to women, men are more likely to use cannabis. Approximately 1 in 25 women in the United States reports using marijuana while pregnant. Research shows that women enter treatment for cannabis use disorder earlier than men (telescoping), but there have been no specific guidelines published regarding gender differences, and its effectiveness of treatment with cannabis use disorder. Some studies suggest that cannabis use is related to premenstrual syndrome and premenstrual dysphoric disorder.

Synthetic Cannabinoid

Synthetic cannabinoid gained its popularity in the U.S.A. in 2008; while it emerged for sale in Europe in 2005. In recent years, they have emerged as drugs of abuse. Synthetic cannabinoids are difficult to detect as it's a mixture of different synthetic chemicals that are sprayed onto leaves. About hundreds of different synthetic cannabinoids were reported in 2014 and more are identified since. They are called Cannabinoids, because of their mechanism of action; both synthetic cannabinoids and cannabis act on the same brain cell receptors the cannabinoid recepter1 (CB1). There is a large misconception of its safety, by the general population. It is readily available, and is about five dollars per bag, and is usually marked as "not for human consumption". Some of the common names are: "K2", "Spice", "Black Mamba", "AK-47", "Bombay Blue", "Mr. Happy", "Scooby Snax", "Genie", "Kush", "Zohai", "Kronic". The CDC identified methods of use as; sprayed onto plant material and smoked, mixed into a liquid, vaped in electronic nicotine delivery devices, or added to herbal tea or to food and consumed.

Men have been identified to use it more than women. Mostly younger age groups consumes this product. According to the Substance Abuse and

Mental Health Service Administration (SAMSHA) 2014 report, there were 28,531 emergency room visits related to synthetic cannabinoids; 30% were females and 70% were males; 78% were adolescents and young adults aged between ages 12-29.

Toxicity with synthetic cannabis are identified as; agitation, sleepiness, irritability, confusion, dizziness, delirium, stroke, seizures, hallucinations, delusions, violent behavior, suicidal thoughts, tachypnea, tachycardia, hypertension, severe nausea, vomiting, chest pain, myocardial infarction, rhabdomyolysis, kidney failure, and death. Commonly reported withdrawal symptoms are reported as; headache, severe anxiety, sweating, trouble sleeping, nausea, vomiting, seizures, rapid heart rate, chest pain, palpitations, and difficulty breathing. Clinical diagnosis is challenging as it does not have any well-defined toxicological syndrome. The typically used urine toxicology does not include synthetic cannabinoids. There are several factors why a facility may not routinely order this screening test, one it's expensive and not always identified secondary to its multiple subtypes of chemicals. Some commercial laboratories offer testing for different synthetic cannabinoids, but might not detect all; results are often delayed. Clinically identifying it in toxicology reports routinely will not change the management of the medical or psychiatric supportive treatment. The patient will usually self-reports its use. Treatment is always supportive. Benzodiazepines are used to treat agitation, combativeness, and muscular hyperactivity, if medically appropriate.

Comorbidities Associated with Cannabis Use

Cannabis intoxication may lead to; delirium, anxiety disorder, psychotic disorder, flashbacks, cognitive impairment, and amotivational syndrome.

CANNABIS USE AND PREGNANCY

There have been very few studies regarding how cannabis affects women and the fetus; CDC recommends against using marijuana during pregnancy. Some research showed correlation between cannabis use and low birth weight and developmental problems. Tetrahydrocannabinol (THC), one of the psychoactive ingredients of cannabis is stored in fat tissue, and limited evidence show that it can be passed on to the new born through breast milk.

TREATMENT FOR THC

Very few studies have been conducted on the effective treatment in women; most of the studies were done in men. The treatment include: Cognitive Behavioral Therapy (CBT), Oral Dronabinol (a synthetic THC) approved by FDA (for anorexia, chemo-related nausea, vomiting, etc.), and Nefazodone.

STIMULANT USE AND WOMEN'S HEALTH

Some known stimulants are: amphetamine, methamphetamine, cocaine, and khat (Leaves of *Catha edulis*) which is found in East Africa. Recent studies have suggested a rise in stimulant use in women whom may be particularly vulnerable to the reinforcing effects of stimulant drugs. Some studies reported increased subjective feelings of high and increased heart rate during the follicular phase, when levels of estrogen are high and progesterone levels are low. According to National Institute of Health, about 5 percent of pregnant women use one or more addictive substances. There have been approximately 750,000 cocaine-exposed pregnancies every year.

Medical Risks with Stimulant in Women

There is a relatively low known risk, of having a baby born with specific defects after taking medications prescribed for Attention Deficit Hyperactivity Disorder treatment. Some studies have suggested increase risk for Gastroschisis, Omphalocele and Transverse Limb Deficiency in newborns. Cocaine use during pregnancy is associated with maternal migraines, seizures, hypertensive crises, premature membrane rupture, spontaneous miscarriage, preterm labor, and difficult delivery.

Treatment for Stimulant Addiction

The treatment is known to be limited, as no prescription is approved, but can be successful with motivational interviewing, cognitive behavioral therapy, and therapeutic community programs.

Benzodiazepines

There is a steady increase of use of benzodiazepines since 1999. Benzodiazepines modulate GABA activity. It is teratogen; and its use in pregnancy is not advised. Use in 3rd trimester can precipitate withdrawal syndrome in newborn. It is secreted in breast milk resulting in dyspnea, bradycardia and drowsiness in newborns.

Recent Canadian study published on May 15th 2019, in Journal of the American Medical Association (JAMA) Psychiatry; reported ‘Benzodiazepine use in early pregnancy is associated with increased risk for spontaneous abortion”. The researchers included “27,000 cases of spontaneous abortion occurring between the 6th and 19th week of gestation with 134,000 control pregnancies. Rates of benzodiazepine use by prescription fills were significantly higher among spontaneous abortion cases than controls (1.4% vs. 0.6%).” This study also noted that higher dose of benzodiazepines was significant associated with higher risk in respect to spontaneous abortion rates. Recommendation based on the study was to use the benzodiazepines if needed, for a shorter duration of time.

Benzodiazepine Induced Disorders

Some serious known sequelae of using, or misusing benzodiazepines, are described as follows; this is whether it is prescribed or not; delirium, respiratory compromise, amnestic disorder, mood disorder, and psychotic disorder.

Signs and Symptoms of Benzodiazepine Withdrawal

Frequently seen signs of withdrawal include: anxiety, irritability, insomnia, tachycardia, hyperreflexia, difficulty in concentrations, seizure, tremor, myoclonus, hyperacusis, depersonalization, and delirium.

Guideline for Treatment of Benzodiazepine Withdrawal

Evaluate medical and psychiatric conditions; with a detailed history. Hospitalize if necessary. Like with ethanol, severe benzodiazepine use, may lead to severe seizures, and or death, if untreated in a timely manner. This warrants admission to detoxification facility or even intensive care unit. Some recommends stabilizing with long acting benzodiazepine while others recommend stabilizing on the same drug or on phenobarbital. Slow tapering to avoid withdrawal is warranted. Psychosocial intervention may be needed.

Treatment of Benzodiazepine Overdose

Monitoring is extremely important in overdose and should include: vital signs, central nervous system activity, gastric lavage, activated charcoal. Antidote option is flumazenil.

Tobacco Use in Women

There are several types of tobacco products, such as cigarettes, cigars, cigarillos, or filtered little cigars, electronic cigarettes (E-cigarettes), smokeless tobacco, pipes, water pipes, or hookahs. According to CDC, almost 34 million adults in the United States smoke cigarette and about 12 of every 100 adult women smoke (12.2%). As per American Cancer Society Lung cancer, both small cell and non-small cell are the 2nd most common cancer in both men and women. (Prostate Cancer in Men and Breast Cancer in women are most common, gender related causes of cancer). About 13% of all new cancers are lung cancers. Lung cancer is by far the leading cause of cancer death among both men and women; more people die of lung cancer than of colon, breast, and prostate cancers combined. Women may have more difficulty quitting smoking. Some data suggest that women are more likely to succeed in quitting smoking during follicular phase of the menstrual cycle compared to luteal phase. Women are more concerned about weight gain related to smoking cessation than men. This fact, contributes to relapse 3 times more often than with men. Tobacco has been associated with premature ovarian failure, hence early menopause.

Cigarette Smoking during Pregnancy

According to CDC in 2011, approximately 10% of women reported smoking during the last 3 months of pregnancy. Of women who smoked 3 months before pregnancy, 55% quit during pregnancy. Among women who quit smoking during pregnancy, 40% started smoking again within 6 months after delivery. Spontaneous abortion, placental separation, premature delivery, low birth weight, Sudden Infant Death Syndrome (SIDS), cleft lip and or cleft palate, newborns with persistent pulmonary hypertension are some of the severe teratogenic effects.

TREATMENT

Nicotine Replacement Therapy (NRT) (more effective for men than women). This includes; bupropion and varenicline which are equally effective both in men and women. Some prefer bupropion in women, because of its antidepressant property. Therapy and counseling are crucial for support, as relapse is as high as 95%.

Table 1. Summary of Treatment Inpatient and Outpatient

Substance	**Inpatient Treatment**	**Outpatient treatment**
Opiate	Buprenorphine with and without naloxone Methadone Clonidine	Buprenorphine with and without naloxone Methadone Long acting intramuscular Naltrexone
Alcohol	Chlordiazepoxide Lorazepam Diazepam	Disulfiram Naltrexone (Oral, Injectable) Acamprosate
Cannabis	Rehabilitation setting individual and group counseling	CBT Oral Dronabinol Nefazodone
Stimulant	Rehabilitation setting individual and group counseling	CBT Therapeutic community program
Benzodiazepine	Long and medium acting Benzodiazepine Phenobarbital. Flumazenil (for acute intoxication)	Psychological intervention -Outpatient Rehabilitation setting individual and group counseling
Tobacco	Rehabilitation setting individual and group counseling	Nicotine Replacement Therapy (NRT) Bupropion, Varenicline Therapy and counseling

REFERENCES

Abuse, Substance. *"Mental Health Services Administration. 2017. Results from the 2016 National Survey on Drug Use and Health: Detailed Tables."* Rockville, MD: Center for Behavioral Health Statistics and Quality (2017) Retrieved 1/30/19.

Brogly, Susan B., Kelley A. Saia, Alexander Y. Walley, Haomo M. Du, and Paola Sebastiani. "Prenatal buprenorphine versus methadone exposure and neonatal outcomes: Systematic review and meta-analysis." *American Journal of Epidemiology* 180, no. 7 (2014): 673-686. Retrieved 1/30/19.

Bryant, Joanne, Joanne Bryant, Carla Treloar, Joanne Bryant, and Carla Treloar. "The gendered context of initiation to injecting drug use: evidence for women as active initiates." *Drug and alcohol review* 26, no. 3 (2007): 287-293. Retrieved 1/30/19.

Center for Disease Control and prevention/*Excessive Alcohol Use and Risks to Women's Health* (2016) Retrieved 1/30/19.

Center for Disease Control and prevention/*Excessive Alcohol Use and Risks to Women's Health Kaplan and Sadock's Synopsis of Psychiatry: Behavioral Sciences Clinical Psychiatry 11th Edition.*

Center for Substance Abuse Treatment. *"Substance abuse treatment: Addressing the specific needs of women"* (2009) Retrieved 2/1/19.

Greenfield, Shelly F., Sudie E. Back, Katie Lawson, and Kathleen T. Brady. "Substance abuse in women." *Psychiatric Clinics* 33, no. 2 (2010): 339-355.

https://www.whitehouse.gov/briefings-statements/president-donald-j-trumps-initiative-stop-opioid-abuse-reduce-drug-supply-demand-2/. Retrieved 11/5/18

Hudak, Mark L., and Rosemarie C. Tan. "Neonatal drug withdrawal." *Pediatrics* 129, no. 2 (2012): e540-e560.

Olsen, Yngvild. "The CDC guideline on opioid prescribing: rising to the challenge." *JAMA* 315, no. 15 (2016): 1577-1579. Retrieved 1/30/19.

Young, Kelly *"Benzodiazepines Carry Increased Risk for Miscarriage"* https://www.jwatch.org/fw115418/2019/05/16/benzodiazepines-carry-increased-risk-miscarriage published 5/15/19; Retrieved 5/16/19.

About the Editors

Sabina Fink, MD

Primary Editor

Present Position:

Physician in Charge

Northwell Health Outpatient Treatment Center-Addiction Psychiatry

(A Division of Long Island Jewish Medical Center)

Garden City Treatment Center, Garden City, NY, US

Academic Affiliations:

1. Northwell Health, Manhasset, NY, US;
2. The Donald and Barbara Zucker School of Medicine at Hofstra/Northwell, Hempstead, NY, US;
3. Bronx-Care Health System, Icahn School of Medicine at Mount Sinai, New York, NY, US

Dr. Sabina Fink is an Addiction Psychiatrist, currently the physician in charge at Northwell Health Outpatient Treatment Center, a division of Long Island Jewish Medical Center, Garden City. Dr. Fink has been published in numerous articles, book chapters, posters, with media mention which have been published, nationally, and internationally. She has been recognized for outstanding leadership, as well by the American Psychiatric Association Resident Recognition Award for Leadership and Clinical Excellence.

E-mail: Sfink3@northwell.edu

Panagiota Korenis, MD

Co-Editor

Present Position:

Psychiatry Residency Director,
Bronx-Care Health System, New York, NY, US

Academic Affiliations:

1. Bronx-Care Health System,
Icahn School of Medicine at Mount Sinai, New York, NY, US;
2. Albert Einstein College of Medicine, Bronx, NY, US

Dr. Panagiota Korenis is currently the Residency Director and Vice-Chair of Education for Department of Psychiatry at Bronx-Care Health System in New York. She is the Assistant Professor at Albert Einstein College of Medicine. Dr. Korenis has been published in numerous articles and posters, which have been presented, nationally and internationally. She has been recognized as an outstanding faculty mentor by the New York State Psychiatric Association.

INDEX

D

E

F

G

H

I

J

K

L

M

S

T

U

V

W

Y

Z